Technological Advances in Sinus and Skull Base Surgery

Editor

RAJ SINDWANI

OTOLARYNGOLOGIC CLINICS OF NORTH AMERICA

www.oto.theclinics.com

Consulting Editor
SUJANA S. CHANDRASEKHAR

June 2017 • Volume 50 • Number 3

ELSEVIER

1600 John F. Kennedy Boulevard • Suite 1800 • Philadelphia, Pennsylvania, 19103-2899

http://www.oto.theclinics.com

OTOLARYNGOLOGIC CLINICS OF NORTH AMERICA Volume 50, Number 3
June 2017 ISSN 0030-6665, ISBN-13: 978-0-323-53021-7

Editor: Jessica McCool
Developmental Editor: Alison Swety

Otolaryngologic Clinics of North America (ISSN 0030-6665) is published bimonthly by Elsevier, Inc., 360 Park Avenue South, New York, NY 10010-1710. Months of issue are February, April, June, August, October, and December. Business and Editorial Offices: 1600 John F. Kennedy Blvd., Suite 1800, Philadelphia, PA 19103-2899. Customer Service Office: 6277 Sea Harbor Drive, Orlando, FL 32887-4800. Periodicals postage paid at New York, NY and additional mailing offices. Subscription prices are $381.00 per year (US individuals), $803.00 per year (US institutions), $100.00 per year (US student/resident), $500.00 per year (Canadian individuals), $1017.00 per year (Canadian institutions), $556.00 per year (international individuals), $1017.00 per year (international institutions), $270.00 per year (international & Canadian student/resident). Foreign air speed delivery is included in all *Clinics'* subscription prices. All prices are subject to change without notice. **POSTMASTER:** Send address changes to *Otolaryngologic Clinics of North America*, Elsevier Health Sciences Division, Subscription Customer Service, 3251 Riverport Lane, Maryland Heights, MO 63043. **Telephone: 1-800-654-2452 (U.S. and Canada); 314-447-8871 (outside U.S. and Canada). Fax: 314-447-8029. E-mail: journalscustomerservice-usa@elsevier.com (for print support); journalsonlinesupport-usa@elsevier.com (for online support).**

Reprints. For copies of 100 or more of articles in this publication, please contact the Commercial Reprints Department, Elsevier Inc., 360 Park Avenue South, New York, NY 10010-1710. Tel.: 212-633-3874; Fax: 212-633-3820; E-mail: reprints@ elsevier.com.

Otolaryngologic Clinics of North America is also published in Spanish by McGraw-Hill Interamericana Editores S.A., P.O. Box 5-237, 06500 Mexico D.F., Mexico.

Otolaryngologic Clinics of North America is covered in *MEDLINE/PubMed (Index Medicus), Current Contents/Clinical Medicine, Excerpta Medica, BIOSIS, Science Citation Index,* and *ISI/BIOMED.*

PROGRAM OBJECTIVE
The goal of the *Otolaryngologic Clinics of North America* is to provide information on the latest trends in patient management, the newest advances; and provide a sound basis for choosing treatment options in the field of otolaryngology.

LEARNING OBJECTIVES
Upon completion of this activity, participants will be able to:
1. Review the recent evolution of technology in sinus and skull base surgery.
2. Discuss emerging trends in robotics and surgical navigation systems in sinus and skull base surgery.
3. Recognize past and upcoming changes in materials and methods in endoscopic surgery.

ACCREDITATION
The Elsevier Office of Continuing Medical Education (EOCME) is accredited by the Accreditation Council for Continuing Medical Education (ACCME) to provide continuing medical education for physicians.

The EOCME designates this enduring material for a maximum of 15 *AMA PRA Category 1 Credit*(s)™. Physicians should claim only the credit commensurate with the extent of their participation in the activity.

All other health care professionals requesting continuing education credit for this enduring material will be issued a certificate of participation.

DISCLOSURE OF CONFLICTS OF INTEREST
The EOCME assesses conflict of interest with its instructors, faculty, planners, and other individuals who are in a position to control the content of CME activities. All relevant conflicts of interest that are identified are thoroughly vetted by EOCME for fair balance, scientific objectivity, and patient care recommendations. EOCME is committed to providing its learners with CME activities that promote improvements or quality in health care and not a specific proprietary business or a commercial interest.

The planning committee, staff, authors and editors listed below have identified no financial relationships or relationships to products or devices they or their spouse/life partner have with commercial interest related to the content of this CME activity:
Omar H. Ahmed, MD; Andre Beer-Furlan, MD; Ricardo L. Carrau, MD; Juanita Celix, MD; Srikant Chakravarthi, MD; Sujana S. Chandrasekhar, MD; Garret W. Choby, MD; Brian D'Anza, MD; John M. DelGaudio, MD; Anjali Fortna; Melanie B. Fukui, MD; Lior Gonen, MD; Ralph Abi Hachem, MD; Ashleigh A. Halderman, MD; Leah J. Hauser, MD; Peter H. Hwang, MD; Joseph B. Jacobs, MD; Jonathan Jennings, MD; Sammy Khalili, MD; Andrew P. Lane, MD; Richard A. Lebowitz, MD; Brian C. Lobo, MD; Lauren J. Luk, MD; Sonya Marcus, MD; Conner J. Massey, MD; Jessica McCool; Alejandro Monroy-Sosa, MD; Premkumar Nandhakumar; Enver Ozer, MD; John F. Pallanch, MD, MS; Daniel Prevedello, MD; Sanjeet Rangarajan, MD, MEng; Richard A. Rovin, MD; Aaron C. Sigler, DO, MS; Raj Sindwani, MD, FACS; Ameet Singh, MD; Janalee K. Stokken, MD; Alison Swety; Dennis Tang, MD; Jonathan Y. Ting, MD, MS, MBA; Dominic Vernon, MD; Sarika Walia, MD; Katie Widmeier; William Yao, MD.

The planning committee, staff, authors and editors listed below have identified financial relationships or relationships to products or devices they or their spouse/life partner have with commercial interest related to the content of this CME activity:
Rakesh K. Chandra, MD is a consultant/advisor for, with research support from, Intersect ENT, Inc.
Martin J. Citardi, MD is a consultant/advisor for Acclarent, Inc.; Biosense Webster, Inc, Part of the Johnson & Johnson Family of Companies; Medical Metrics; and Medtronic.
Amin B. Kassam, MD is a consultant/advisor for Synaptive Medical and Medtronic, and has royalties/patents from KLS Martin Group.
Amber Luong, MD, PhD is a consultant/advisor for 480 Biomedical; Aerin Medical Inc; Medtronic; Medical Metrics; and ENTvantage Inc, and has stock ownership in ENTvantage Inc.
Pablo F. Recinos, MD is a consultant/advisor for, with stock ownership in, Acera Surgical Inc.
Justin H. Turner, MD, PhD is a consultant/advisor for Intersect ENT, Inc.
Troy D. Woodard, MD is a consultant/advisor for Acclarent, Inc. and Intersect ENT, Inc.

UNAPPROVED/OFF-LABEL USE DISCLOSURE
The EOCME requires CME faculty to disclose to the participants:
1. When products or procedures being discussed are off-label, unlabelled, experimental, and/or investigational (not US Food and Drug Administration [FDA] approved); and
2. Any limitations on the information presented, such as data that are preliminary or that represent ongoing research, interim analyses, and/or unsupported opinions. Faculty may discuss information about

pharmaceutical agents that is outside of FDA-approved labelling. This information is intended solely for CME and is not intended to promote off-label use of these medications. If you have any questions, contact the medical affairs department of the manufacturer for the most recent prescribing information.

TO ENROLL

To enroll in the *Otolaryngologic Clinics of North America* Continuing Medical Education program, call customer service at 1-800-654-2452 or sign up online at http://www.theclinics.com/home/cme. The CME program is available to subscribers for an additional annual fee of USD 260.

METHOD OF PARTICIPATION

In order to claim credit, participants must complete the following:
1. Complete enrolment as indicated above.
2. Read the activity.
3. Complete the CME Test and Evaluation. Participants must achieve a score of 70% on the test. All CME Tests and Evaluations must be completed online.

CME INQUIRIES/SPECIAL NEEDS

For all CME inquiries or special needs, please contact elsevierCME@elsevier.com.

Contributors

CONSULTING EDITOR

SUJANA S. CHANDRASEKHAR, MD
Director, New York Otology, Clinical Professor of Otolaryngology–Head and Neck Surgery, Hofstra-Northwell School of Medicine, Clinical Associate Professor of Otolaryngology–Head and Neck Surgery, Icahn School of Medicine at Mount Sinai, New York, New York; Past President, American Academy of Otolaryngology–Head and Neck Surgery, Alexandria, Virginia

EDITOR

RAJ SINDWANI, MD, FACS
Vice Chairman and Head, Section of Rhinology, Sinus and Skull Base Surgery, Head and Neck Institute, Co-Director, Minimally Invasive Cranial Base and Pituitary Surgery Program, Head and Neck Institute, Rose Ella Burkhardt Brain Tumor and Neuro-Oncology Center, Cleveland Clinic, Cleveland, Ohio

AUTHORS

OMAR H. AHMED, MD
Resident Physician, Department of Otolaryngology–Head and Neck Surgery, New York University, New York, New York

ANDRE BEER-FURLAN, MD
Clinical Fellow in Skull Base Surgery, Department of Neurological Surgery, The Ohio State University Wexner Medical Center, Columbus, Ohio

RICARDO L. CARRAU, MD
Professor, Department of Otolaryngology–Head and Neck Surgery, Director of the Comprehensive Skull Base Surgery Program, The Ohio State University Wexner Medical Center, Columbus, Ohio

JUANITA CELIX, MD
St. Luke's Medical Center, Aurora Neuroscience Innovation Institute, Milwaukee, Wisconsin

SRIKANT CHAKRAVARTHI, MD
St. Luke's Medical Center, Aurora Neuroscience Innovation Institute, Milwaukee, Wisconsin

RAKESH K. CHANDRA, MD
Professor of Otolaryngology–Head and Neck Surgery, Chief, Rhinology, Sinus and Skull Base Surgery, Vanderbilt University, Nashville, Tennessee

GARRET W. CHOBY, MD
Division of Rhinology and Skull Base Surgery, Department of Otolaryngology–Head and Neck Surgery, Stanford University, Stanford, California

MARTIN J. CITARDI, MD
Professor and Chair, Department of Otorhinolaryngology–Head and Neck Surgery, McGovern Medical School, The University of Texas Health Science Center at Houston, Houston, Texas

BRIAN D'ANZA, MD
Assistant Professor, Section of Rhinology, Sinus and Skull Base Surgery, Department of Otolaryngology, University Hospitals–Case Western Reserve University, Cleveland, Ohio

JOHN M. DELGAUDIO, MD
Vice Chair, Gerald S. Gussack Professor of Otolaryngology, Chief of Rhinology and Sinus Surgery, Department of Otolaryngology–Head and Neck Surgery, Emory University, Atlanta, Georgia

MELANIE B. FUKUI, MD
St. Luke's Medical Center, Aurora Neuroscience Innovation Institute, Milwaukee, Wisconsin

LIOR GONEN, MD
St. Luke's Medical Center, Aurora Neuroscience Innovation Institute, Milwaukee, Wisconsin

RALPH ABI HACHEM, MD
Assistant Professor, Division of Head and Neck Surgery and Communication Sciences, Department of Surgery, Duke University Medical Center, Durham, North Carolina

ASHLEIGH A. HALDERMAN, MD
Assistant Professor, Department of Otolaryngology–Head and Neck Surgery, University of Texas Southwestern Medical Center, Dallas, Texas

LEAH J. HAUSER, MD
Clinical Instructor of Otolaryngology–Head and Neck Surgery, Fellow, Rhinology, Sinus and Skull Base Surgery, Vanderbilt University, Nashville, Tennessee

PETER H. HWANG, MD
Division of Rhinology and Skull Base Surgery, Department of Otolaryngology–Head and Neck Surgery, Stanford University, Stanford, California

JOSEPH B. JACOBS, MD
Professor, Department of Otolaryngology–Head and Neck Surgery, New York University, New York, New York

JONATHAN JENNINGS, MD
St. Luke's Medical Center, Aurora Neuroscience Innovation Institute, Milwaukee, Wisconsin

AMIN B. KASSAM, MD
St. Luke's Medical Center, Aurora Neuroscience Innovation Institute, Milwaukee, Wisconsin

SAMMY KHALILI, MD
St. Luke's Medical Center, Aurora Neuroscience Innovation Institute, Milwaukee, Wisconsin

ANDREW P. LANE, MD
Professor, Department of Otolaryngology–Head and Neck Surgery, Johns Hopkins School of Medicine, Baltimore, Maryland

RICHARD A. LEBOWITZ, MD
Associate Professor, Department of Otolaryngology–Head and Neck Surgery, New York University, New York, New York

BRIAN C. LOBO, MD
Fellow, Section of Rhinology, Sinus and Endoscopic Skull Base Surgery, Department of Otolaryngology–Head and Neck Surgery, Head and Neck Institute, Cleveland Clinic, Cleveland, Ohio

LAUREN J. LUK, MD
Rhinology Fellow, Department of Otolaryngology–Head and Neck Surgery, Emory University, Atlanta, Georgia

AMBER LUONG, MD, PhD
Department of Otorhinolaryngology–Head and Neck Surgery, McGovern Medical School, The University of Texas Health Science Center at Houston, Houston, Texas

SONYA MARCUS, MD
Resident Physician, Department of Otolaryngology–Head and Neck Surgery, New York University, New York, New York

CONNER J. MASSEY, MD
Resident Physician, Department of Otolaryngology, University of Colorado School of Medicine, Aurora, Colorado

ALEJANDRO MONROY-SOSA, MD
St. Luke's Medical Center, Aurora Neuroscience Innovation Institute, Milwaukee, Wisconsin

ENVER OZER, MD
Professor, Department of Otolaryngology–Head and Neck Surgery, The Ohio State University Wexner Medical Center, Columbus, Ohio

JOHN F. PALLANCH, MD, MS
Emeritus, Department of Otorhinolaryngology, Mayo Clinic, Rochester, Minnesota

DANIEL PREVEDELLO, MD
Associate Professor, Department of Neurological Surgery, The Ohio State University Wexner Medical Center, Columbus, Ohio

SANJEET RANGARAJAN, MD, MEng
Adjunct Assistant Professor, Department of Otolaryngology–Head and Neck Surgery, The Ohio State University Wexner Medical Center, Columbus, Ohio

PABLO F. RECINOS, MD
Minimally Invasive Cranial Base and Pituitary Surgery Program, Section of Rhinology, Sinus and Skull Base Surgery, Head and Neck Institute, Rose Ella Burkhardt Brain Tumor and Neuro-Oncology Center, Cleveland Clinic, Cleveland, Ohio

RICHARD A. ROVIN, MD
St. Luke's Medical Center, Aurora Neuroscience Innovation Institute, Milwaukee, Wisconsin

AARON C. SIGLER, DO, MS
Tulane Center for Clinical Neurosciences, Department of Neurosurgery, New Orleans, Louisiana

RAJ SINDWANI, MD, FACS
Vice Chairman and Head, Section of Rhinology, Sinus and Skull Base Surgery, Head and Neck Institute, Co-Director, Minimally Invasive Cranial Base and Pituitary Surgery Program, Head and Neck Institute, Rose Ella Burkhardt Brain Tumor and Neuro-Oncology Center, Cleveland Clinic, Cleveland, Ohio

AMEET SINGH, MD
Associate Professor of Surgery, Director, Rhinology and Skull Base Surgery, Division of Otolaryngology–Head and Neck Surgery, The George Washington University School of Medicine, Washington, DC

JANALEE K. STOKKEN, MD
Assistant Professor of Otolaryngology, Department of Otorhinolaryngology, Mayo Clinic, Rochester, Minnesota

DENNIS TANG, MD
Section of Rhinology and Skull Base Surgery, Minimally Invasive Cranial Base and Pituitary Surgery Program, Head and Neck Institute, Rose Ella Burkhardt Brain Tumor and Neuro-Oncology Center, Cleveland Clinic, Cleveland, Ohio

JONATHAN Y. TING, MD, MS, MBA
Assistant Professor, Department of Otolaryngology–Head and Neck Surgery, Indiana University School of Medicine, Indiana University, Indianapolis, Indiana

JUSTIN H. TURNER, MD, PhD
Associate Professor of Otolaryngology–Head and Neck Surgery, Rhinology, Sinus and Skull Base Surgery, Vanderbilt University, Nashville, Tennessee

DOMINIC VERNON, MD
Resident, Department of Otolaryngology–Head and Neck Surgery, Indiana University School of Medicine, Indiana University, Indianapolis, Indiana

SARIKA WALIA, MD
St. Luke's Medical Center, Aurora Neuroscience Innovation Institute, Milwaukee, Wisconsin

TROY D. WOODARD, MD
Minimally Invasive Cranial Base and Pituitary Surgery Program, Attending Staff Surgeon, Section of Rhinology, Sinus and Skull Base Surgery, Head and Neck Institute, Rose Ella Burkhardt Brain Tumor and Neuro-Oncology Center, Cleveland Clinic, Cleveland, Ohio

WILLIAM YAO, MD
Assistant Professor, Department of Otorhinolaryngology–Head and Neck Surgery, McGovern Medical School, The University of Texas Health Science Center at Houston, Houston, Texas

Contents

Rhinoscopy became a formal field of study in the mid-nineteenth century as improvements in nasal specula were made and the potent vasoconstrictive effects of cocaine on the intranasal tissues were discovered. Since then, a multitude of advances in visualization and illumination have been made. The advent of the Storz-Hopkins endoscope in the mid-twentieth century represents a culmination of efforts spanning nearly 2 centuries, and illumination has evolved concomitantly. The future of endoscopic sinus surgery may integrate developing technologies, such as 3-dimensional endoscopy, augmented reality navigation systems, and robotic endoscope holders.

Modern advances in DNA sequencing have allowed for the development of culture-independent techniques with application to infectious and inflammatory conditions, such as rhinosinusitis. Although paradigm-changing discoveries have resulted from molecular microbiologic methods for a number of diseases, insights provided into the role of bacteria in chronic rhinosinusitis have yet to be fully understood to the point of impacting clinical diagnosis and management. As culture-independent techniques continue to evolve and become more refined, it is likely that a better understanding will emerge of how the microbiome influences chronic rhinosinusitis pathogenesis and response to therapy.

Chronic rhinosinusitis is recognized as an inflammatory syndrome involving the nose and paranasal sinuses of multifactorial etiology. Research has demonstrated a complex interplay between host factors, microbiota, environmental exposures, and epigenetics resulting in chronic mucosal inflammation. The mainstay of medical therapy addresses this inflammation. In previously operated sinuses this includes topical saline and corticosteroids, reserving antibiotics for culture-directed acute exacerbations. Topical antiinflammatory therapies allow increased local concentration of drugs while minimizing side effects. Topical therapies have advanced the surgical field by improving and maintaining postoperative outcomes. The topical therapies include saline, corticosteroids, antibiotics, and antifungals.

Nasal biomaterials have been developed to improve postoperative outcomes after functional endoscopic sinus surgery (FESS). These products have been designed to overcome certain common complications in FESS, and to maximize patient comfort. This article evaluates the performance of nonabsorbable and absorbable packing with respect to these outcomes. The collected trials suggest superior performance of bioabsorbable packs compared with absorbable packs with respect to patient comfort. For hemostasis and wound healing, variation in performance metrics makes interstudy comparison difficult. Before further trials are conducted, consensus must be reached among rhinologists as to the proper method of evaluating these products.

Stenting has long been used in the paranasal sinuses with the goals of maintaining a patent sinus cavity during the postoperative healing process and preventing restenosis from inflammation or scarring. More recently, drug-eluting stents have been introduced. Steroid-impregnated dressings and implants appear to be safe, although likely have increased systemic absorption compared with topical nasal steroid sprays and rinses. There is evidence to support the use of steroid-releasing implants in the ethmoid cavity in the postoperative period; however, more study is needed to truly define the role of these implants.

Since being introduced more than 10 years ago, balloon catheter technology (BCT) has undergone several generations of innovations. From construction to utilization, there has been a myriad of advancements in balloon technology. The ergonomics of the balloon dilation systems have improved with a focus on limiting the extra assembly. "Hybrid" BCT procedures have shown promise in mucosal preservation, including treating isolated complex frontal disease. Multiple randomized clinical trials report improved long-term outcomes in stand-alone BCT, including in-office use. The ever-expanding technological innovations ensure BCT will be a key component in the armamentarium of the modern sinus surgeon.

Nasal septal perforations, particularly those that are large and irregular in shape, often present as challenging surgical dilemmas. New technology has allowed us to develop techniques using computed tomography imaging and 3-dimensional (3D) printers to design custom polymeric silicone septal buttons. These buttons offer patients an option that avoids a surgical intervention when standard buttons do not fit well or are not tolerated. Preliminary data suggest that buttons designed by 3D printer technology provide more comfort than standard commercially available or hand-carved buttons with equivalent reduction of symptoms.

Since its application in nasal surgery, the microdebrider has revolutionized the practice of endoscopic sinus surgery. As the demands and breadth of procedures performed endoscopically have increased, so has the need for improvement in the microdebrider and related technologies. This article addresses how use of the microdebrider has impacted endonasal surgery and discusses current advances, which include creation of specialty hand pieces and blades, increases in instrument rotational speed, incorporation of navigation and energy, adaptation for intracranial use, and disposable instrumentation designed for in office use. Advances in microdebrider technology have improved functionality and expanded the utility of these devices.

Coblation is a technology that incorporates bipolar radiofrequency energy to ablate tissue at relatively low temperatures. Its use for sinonasal surgery is actively being investigated, including applications for turbinate reduction, sinus surgery, skull base surgery, and adenoidectomy. Potential benefits include reduction in blood loss, improved endoscopic surgical visualization, and reduction in postoperative pain. The main drawbacks are its relatively high cost, potential adverse effects on functional epithelium, and relative paucity of long-term outcomes.

Ultrasonic aspirators (UAs) are increasingly being used in rhinology and skull base surgery. The use of ultrasonic vibration for the removal of bony tissue transfers minimal heat to surrounding tissues and is relatively atraumatic to nearby soft tissue structures. This article details the development and application of this technology in septoturbinoplasty, endoscopic dacryocystorhinostomy (DCR), and skull base surgery. The benefits and limitations of UAs compared with conventionally powered instruments are discussed.

Over the past 25 years, rhinologists have adopted surgical navigation technology for endoscopic sinus and skull base procedures. Navigation systems often produce a wide target registration error (TRE). Ideally, next-generation systems will include a leap in target registration error reduce TRE through innovative hardware and software. Incorporation of microsensors will be another important innovation. Future systems are likely to include augmented reality, which can project overlays of critical anatomy on real-world endoscopic images. Recent trends in surgical navigation suggest a phase of rapid evolution.

Transoral robotic surgery (TORS) has been proven to be safe and to yield acceptable oncological and functional outcomes for surgery of the oropharynx, hypopharynx, supraglottis, and glottis. TORS has been successful at reducing morbidity, improving quality of life, and providing access to areas that previously required mandibulotomy or other more radical approaches in the past. This has changed the paradigm of management of tumors in these anatomic locations. In this article, the authors review the recent literature discussing the role of robotic surgery in managing sinonasal and skull base pathology and discuss its current advantages and limitations.

Endoscopic skull base surgery has developed rapidly over the last decade, in large part because of the expanding armamentarium of endoscopic repair techniques. This article reviews the available technologies and techniques, including vascularized and nonvascularized flaps, synthetic grafts, sealants and glues, and multilayer reconstruction. Understanding which of these repair methods is appropriate and under what circumstances is paramount to achieving success in this challenging but rewarding field. A graduated approach to skull base reconstruction is presented to provide a systematic framework to guide selection of repair technique to ensure a successful outcome while minimizing morbidity for the patient.

 Video content accompanies this article at http://www.oto.theclinics. com.

Technological advancement in the operating room is evolving into a dynamic system mirroring that of the aeronautics industry. Through data visualization, information is continuously being captured, collected, and stored on a scalable informatics platform for rapid, intuitive, iterative learning. The authors believe this philosophy (paradigm) will feed into an intelligent informatics domain fully accessible to all and geared toward precision, cell-based therapy in which tissue can be targeted and interrogated in situ. In future, the operating room will be a venue that facilitates this real-time tissue interrogation, which will guide in situ therapeutics to restore the state of health.

OTOLARYNGOLOGIC CLINICS
OF NORTH AMERICA

RELATED INTEREST

Radiologic Clinics
January 2017 (Vol. 55, Issue 1)
Skull Base Imaging
Nafi Aygun, *Editor*
Available at: http://www.radiologic.theclinics.com

THE CLINICS ARE AVAILABLE ONLINE!
Access your subscription at:
www.theclinics.com

Retraction

The article, "Laryngeal Function After Radiation Therapy," by Mauricio Gamez, Kenneth Hu, and Louis B. Harrison, originally published in the August 2015 issue of *Otolaryngologic Clinics* (Volume 48, Issue 4, pp. 585–599), has been retracted. Please see the Elsevier Policy on Article Withdrawal (http://www.elsevier.com/locate/withdrawalpolicy).

This article has been retracted at the request of the Editors.

The authors realized after publication that parts of this paper had not been properly rewritten and cited before submission of the final article to the publisher. Parts of this paper have already appeared in Curr Oncol Rep (2012) 14:158–165. DOI http://dx.doi.org/10.1007/s11912-012-0216-1. The authors of this paper apologize to the authors of the original paper, the scientific community, and to readers of the journal that this was not detected at the manuscript submission stage.

Otolaryngol Clin N Am 50 (2017) xv
http://dx.doi.org/10.1016/j.otc.2017.03.001
0030-6665/17/© 2017 Elsevier Inc. All rights reserved.

oto.theclinics.com

Foreword

Harnessing Technology at the Edges of Otolaryngology

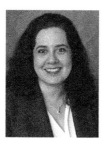

Sujana S. Chandrasekhar, MD
Consulting Editor

The first frontal sinus surgery was described in 1750 by Runge, who performed an obliteration procedure. An external and intracranial drainage procedure for a frontal sinus mucocele was described in 1870, and in 1884, the era of trephination was born (Ogston-Luc procedure), but abandoned due to the high rate of nasofrontal duct stenosis and surgical failure. Radical ablation procedures with removal of the anterior table and mucosal stripping were introduced in 1895, but because of the significant cosmetic deformity and high failure rates, conservative procedures became de rigeur from 1905 onward. The most famous of these was the Lothrop procedure of combined intranasal and external ethmoidectomy and resection of the sinus floor, superior nasal septum, and frontal sinus septum. This was dangerous due to lack of visualization during the intranasal approach, and, unfortunately, continued to result in orbital soft tissue prolapse into the ethmoid area and restenosis of the frontal drainage pathway. External frontoethmoidectomy began in Germany at the turn of the 20th century and was popularized in the United States by Lynch and in the United Kingdom by Howarth in the early 1920s. Failure rates of up to 33% resulted in modifications of the procedure, but long-term failure rates remained up to 30%. Osteoplastic anterior wall approaches to the frontal sinus had been described over 150 years prior, but it was not until the 1950s that successful reports with no complications and no cosmetic deformity were reported in the literature; this technique became the standard in the 1960s and onward for several decades. In the 1990s, the problem of poor visualization was solved with the introduction of endoscopic and microscopic approaches to the sinuses, including the frontal sinus.[1] This adaptation of technology changed a difficult, disfiguring, relatively unsuccessful surgical challenge into one that could be adopted and used in a widespread fashion.

Dr Raj Sindwani has compiled a comprehensive review of the many technological advances in sinus and skull base surgery in this issue of *Otolaryngologic Clinics of North America*. Those of us who bridged training between "blind" intranasal sinus

Otolaryngol Clin N Am 50 (2017) xvii–xviii
http://dx.doi.org/10.1016/j.otc.2017.03.003
0030-6665/17/© 2017 Published by Elsevier Inc.

surgery and endoscopic techniques will appreciate the evolution in visualization that enables current surgeons to approach not only sinus disease but also disease at the anterior skull base with confidence. That change was equivalent to the change from black-and-white Kansas to technicolor Oz in the movie *The Wizard of Oz*. But that is not the only technological breakthrough addressed here. Our understanding of the microbiome in chronic rhinosinusitis enables targeted topical therapies and the use of absorbable and drug-eluting materials safely. Using microdebriders and ultrasonic aspirators is a far cry and significant advancement from bloody removal of polypoid nasal tissue using a cups forceps through a nasal speculum. In complex and revision cases, the advent of surgical navigation and use of robotic technology will enable aggressive yet safe surgical management. Reconstruction of that all-important floor between the intracranial cavity and the nose/sinuses, and doing so endoscopically, highlights technological advancements that are truly life-saving. And the look at the future, with the incorporation of three-dimensional printing and designing futuristic operating rooms, shows what can be.

I congratulate the authors of each section on their forward-thinking exploration of each subject, and Dr Sindwani on selecting the topics and the authors, and putting this issue of *Otolaryngologic Clinics of North America* together.

Sujana S. Chandrasekhar, MD
Director, New York Otology
Departments of Otolaryngology-Head and Neck Surgery
Hofstra-Northwell School of Medicine
Icahn School of Medicine at Mount Sinai
1421 Third Avenue, 4th Floor
New York, NY 10028, USA

E-mail address:
ssc@nyotology.com

REFERENCE

1. Ramadan HH. History of frontal sinus surgery. Chapter 1. Available at: http://eknygos.lsmuni.lt/springer/166/1-6.pdf. Accessed March 16, 2017.

Preface

Technological Advances in Sinus and Skull Base Surgery

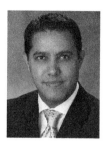

Raj Sindwani, MD, FACS
Editor

Technological advances have always played a major role in the field of Rhinology and Skull Base Surgery. As minimally invasive approaches to the sinuses, orbit, and skull base were developed, pioneering surgeons relied heavily on specialized tools to access and target different anatomic reaches of the head. Since then, technology has continued to evolve in pace with our techniques and areas of focus, with a major emphasis being on multifunctional design and ergonomics. There has been a refinement in foundational tools such as microdebriders that now permit more effective drilling and are cautery enabled; enhancement in our surgical navigation systems that are providing "multimodal" information; and an explosion of bioabsorbable packing materials, including the first ever drug-eluting stent for use in the sinuses.

With the proliferation of endoscopic skull base approaches, we have also experienced a robust expansion in technologies that are sensitive to the narrow confines and environment of exposed neurovital structures characteristic of endonasal skull base and intracranial surgery. Novel devices along with existing platforms with adaptations supportive of intracranial applications have made soft tissue removal, bone removal, and complex skull base reconstruction much more efficacious. Integrated operating rooms and informatics promise to revolutionize the surgeon's interface with the patient and the diseases processes we treat.

The tools that enable us have mirrored the needs of the procedures that we are trying to perform, and more recently they have also helped facilitate *where* we are trying to perform them. With the increased focus on health care spending and costs, we are now seeing a growing trend of minimally invasive procedures moving from the higher-cost operating room environment to the lower-cost in-office setting. This affords benefits to the patient, the surgeon, and indeed the entire health system. Considerations for in-office applications of any technology include being disposable, ease of use (simple setup with intuitive function), multisinus applications, small size and footprint, of course, low cost.

Otolaryngol Clin N Am 50 (2017) xix–xx
http://dx.doi.org/10.1016/j.otc.2017.03.002
oto.theclinics.com

For this project, we asked thought-leaders in the field to vet current technologies in the Rhinology space. They were asked to examine how the technology platform works, to explore its key advantages and limitations, and to comment upon its current and future role. They also examined the literature for the evidence supporting the impact of these devices on disease management and patient outcomes.

It was particularly exciting to work on this issue of *Otolaryngologic Clinics of North America* highlighting technological advancements, as the past decade has witnessed a massive influx of industry funding, innovation, and interest directed to the field of Rhinology. I am personally indebted to my colleagues and friends for their generosity in sharing their insights and expertise, and I hope that the experience shared within this unique issue of *Otolaryngologic Clinics of North America* will be helpful to the reader caring for patients with disorders affecting the sinuses and skull base.

It truly is a great time to be a Rhinologist!

Raj Sindwani, MD, FACS
Rhinology, Sinus and Skull Base Surgery
Head and Neck Institute
Rose Ella Burkhardt Brain Tumor and Neuro-Oncology Center
Cleveland Clinic
Cleveland, OH 44195, USA

E-mail address:
sindwar@ccf.org

Evolution in Visualization for Sinus and Skull Base Surgery

From Headlight to Endoscope

Omar H. Ahmed, MD*, Sonya Marcus, MD,
Richard A. Lebowitz, MD, Joseph B. Jacobs, MD

KEYWORDS

- Rhinoscopy • Fiberoptics • Nasal endoscopy • Endoscope
- Endoscopic sinus surgery • Visualization • Illumination • Historical perspective

KEY POINTS

- The beginnings of rhinoscopy date back to ancient Egypt; however, it was not until the mid-nineteenth century that rhinoscopy emerged as a prominent field of study.
- The evolution of sinonasal endoscopy began with Bozzini's Lichleiter in 1805. Through the innovations of Desormeaux, Nitze, Hirschmann, and Hopkins, the rod-lens endoscope was eventually realized in 1959.
- Advances in illumination replaced antiquated candle light with wire/filament sources.
- The future of endoscopic visualization may entail technologies currently in development, such as 3-dimensional endoscopy, augmented reality navigation systems, and robotic endoscope holders.

Optimizing visualization of the internal nasal structures has been an age-old pursuit bringing forth several instruments, modes of illumination, methods of examination, and technologies. As clear visualization allows for accurate diagnosis and treatment, its importance cannot be overstated. Perhaps the English surgeon and anatomist Thomas Vicary posited this best as he wrote, "The Chirurgeon must knowe the Anatomie, for all authors write against those surgeons that work in man's body not knowing the Anatomie: for they be likened to a blind man that cutteth in a vine tree, for he taketh away more or less than he ought to do."[1]

Financial Disclosures: None.
Department of Otolaryngology–Head and Neck Surgery, New York University, 550 First Avenue - NBV 5E5, New York, NY 10016, USA
* Corresponding author.
E-mail address: Omar.Ahmed@nyumc.org

Otolaryngol Clin N Am 50 (2017) 505–519
http://dx.doi.org/10.1016/j.otc.2017.01.003
0030-6665/17/© 2017 Elsevier Inc. All rights reserved.

THE EARLY HISTORY OF RHINOSCOPY

Study of the nasal cavity and sinuses historically dates back to ancient Egypt (1540–1075 BC) when physicians removed intracranial contents through the nose as part of the mummification process.[2–4] Crude instruments were used and little attention was paid to the intranasal anatomy leading to the cranium. The first major innovation to facilitate visualization of the nasal cavity was the advent of the nasal speculum. Early specula were originally constructed of iron or lead with the purpose of administering medication, cauterization, or protecting intranasal structures during procedures.[4] The first documented intranasal examination was performed by Indian surgeon Sushruta Samhita (circa 600 BC) and reported in an ancient Sanskrit text titled the "Sushruta Samhita" in which he described using a tubular nasal speculum for diagnosis and procedures such as removal of nasal polyps.[3] A crude nasal speculum was also used by Hippocrates (460–370 BC) to cauterize patients with epistaxis. However, it was not until Markusovsky's nasal speculum (**Fig. 1**) in 1859 that semblance of today's nasal speculum emerged.[4,5]

But it was Czermak's invention of a mirror attached to a long shaft to visualize the posterior nasal cavity and nasopharynx from the oropharynx in 1859 that spurred interest in intranasal examination and led to the discovery of the adenoids by Meyer

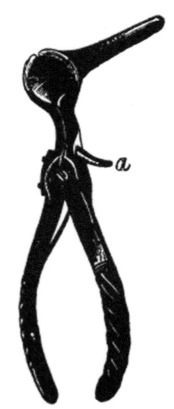

Fig. 1. Markusovsky's nasal speculum. (*From* Baber EC. Chapter IV: Examination of the nose. In: Baber EC, editor. A guide to examination of the nose with remarks on the diagnosis of diseases of the nasal cavities. London: HK Lewis; 1886. p. 57.)

in 1869.[5,6] This device was similar to the laryngeal mirror, which was introduced years earlier in 1855 by singing Professor Manuel Garcia. Czermak termed this new method of examination "rhinoscopy."[4,6] To aid in visualization, palate hooks and various other devices were devised to draw the palate and uvula forward.[7] Markusovsky's nasal speculum and Czermak's mirror for posterior rhinoscopy mark the beginning of modern day rhinoscopy. Interestingly, the latter quickly became popular throughout Europe, whereas little attention was paid to anterior rhinoscopy for nearly a decade.[6]

Only after the introduction of posterior rhinoscopy did significant interest in anterior rhinoscopy arise.[6] In 1868, Thudichum published details on an innovative nasal speculum made of a springlike wiry metal with solid metal blades that widened the nasal vestibule, allowing for improved visualization. He also pointed out the relative neglect of anterior rhinoscopy at the time, which he attributed to lack of proper specula.[4,6] In 1869, Wertheim introduced an instrument similar to the laryngeal mirror but with fenestrae at the end to prevent mucous from obscuring visualization. This device was coined the "conchoscope," as it facilitated view of the lateral nasal wall and turbinates.[7]

A number of subsequent improvements in the nasal speculum were also made, as interest in anterior rhinoscopy continued to grow.[6] Of note, Bernhard Fraenkel from Berlin modified the speculum in 1872 to have fenestrated blades and a central screw for self-retaining (**Fig. 2**).[4,7] To address the difficulty of visualization past the head of the inferior turbinate, Zaufal introduced a funnel-shaped speculum spanning the length of the nasal cavity in 1875.[6,7] Zaufal's speculum eventually became obsolete when the vasoconstrictive effects of cocaine were discovered and its use in the nose and throat were described by Jellinek in 1884.[5,6] Cocaine was used initially in ocular and laryngologic procedures, but was later adopted for use in rhinology where it proved to be invaluable. As a potent vasoconstrictor and anesthetic, it enabled rapid and wide visualization of the nasal cavity, making deeper structures more accessible to direct visualization and instrumentation.[6]

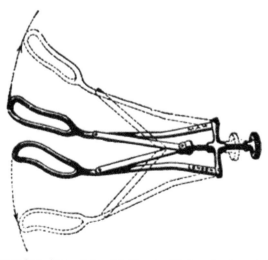

Fig. 2. Fraenkel's speculum. (*From* Baber EC. Chapter IV: Examination of the nose. In: Baber EC, editor. A guide to examination of the nose with remarks on the diagnosis of diseases of the nasal cavities. London: HK Lewis; 1886. p. 50.)

ADVANCES IN ILLUMINATION BEFORE THE FIBEROPTIC ERA

Sufficient illumination was a major challenge in early rhinoscopy.[3] The earliest method of examining the nasal cavity was to tilt the nose upward while the examiner attempted to view the nasal cavity with the aid of sunlight.[4] The use of a light source to visualize the nasal cavity was first described by Aranzi of Bologna in the late sixteenth century as he projected sunlight through a glass flask filled with water.[8] Later, a concave mirror to reflect sunlight into the nasal cavity was developed by Borel.[3] A concave mirror with a central aperture for visualization was introduced in 1841 (**Fig. 3**) by Friedrich Hoffman, an instrument originally intended for otology but subsequently adapted for laryngoscopy and posterior rhinoscopy. His instrument was considered by many to markedly improve visualization and illumination during anterior rhinoscopy.[3–5,9–11] It could be fixed to a headband, spectacle frame, or could be attached to a wooden rod to be held between the surgeon's teeth and was intended to be used with sun or candlelight.[10] This device was largely popularized by John Avery, who used it routinely while indirectly visualizing the larynx with a laryngeal mirror.[11–13] The "head mirror" was further refined in 1868 when Malachia de Cristoforis fixed a small gas lamp below the mirror, improving illumination.

In 1879, Thomas Edison invented the incandescent lamp, enabling laryngologist Alfred Kirstein in the late nineteenth century to modify the head mirror and devise the first electric headlight. It deflected light at a right angle off of a small convex mirror placed inferiorly to the electric bulb, which also contained a small central aperture for visualization.[14–16] Dr Conrad Clar of Austria refined this instrument by outfitting the mirror with 2 lateral apertures instead of only one centrally placed, allowing for stereoscopic vision (**Fig. 4**).[13]

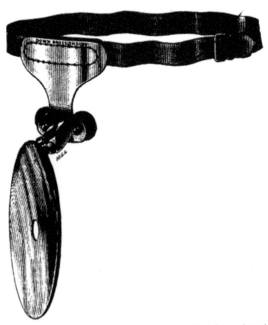

Fig. 3. Head mirror: concave mirror with central aperture fixed to a head band. (*From* Baber EC. Chapter IV: Examination of the nose. In: Baber EC, editor. A guide to examination of the nose with remarks on the diagnosis of diseases of the nasal cavities. London: HK Lewis; 1886. p. 61.)

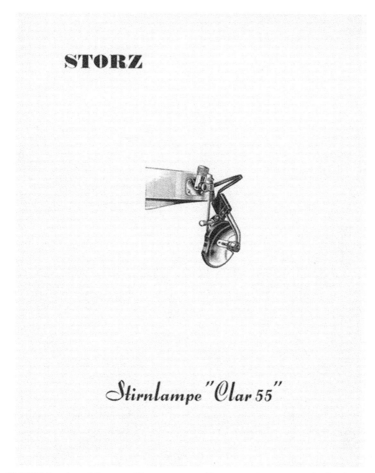

Fig. 4. CLAR55 forehead lamp with concave reflector and tungsten bulb. (©2016 Photo *Courtesy of* KARL STORZ Endoscopy-America, Inc.)

THE ADVENT OF SINONASAL ENDOSCOPY AND FIBEROPTIC ILLUMINATION

An instrument designed to illuminate and visualize the internal structures of the body was first introduced by Philipp Bozzini in 1805. He successfully visualized the human urethra using a device he called the Lichtleiter or "light conductor" (**Fig. 5**). This device consisted of a concave mirror behind a light chamber illuminated by a wax candle that projected light into an aluminum tube. Tubes of various sizes were fashioned for examination of the rectum, urethra, esophagus, and nose.[17] His invention was criticized by the medical faculty of Vienna and regarded as nothing more than a mere "toy."[14,18] Only after his death did his invention generate interest.

French urologist Antonin Jean Desormeaux built on Bozzini's work and in 1853 designed an instrument to examine the urethra and bladder. This device provided continuous illumination from an alcohol and turpentine burning lamp, and used lens to narrow and intensify the field of light. Desormeaux called the device an

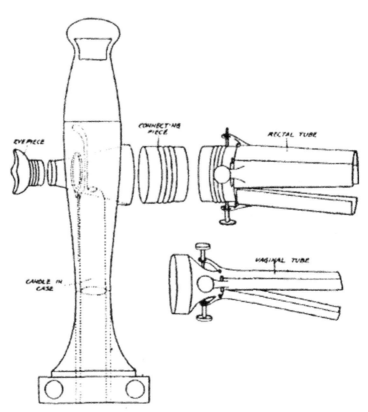

Fig. 5. Lichtleiter with rectal and vaginal tubes. (*From* Moore I. Peroral endoscopy: an historical survey from its origin to the present day. J Laryngol Otol 1926;41:81; with permission.)

"endoscope"(**Fig. 6**), a term not previously used before, and presented it at the Academy in Paris in 1865.[8] Although a refinement from the Lichtleiter, the device continued to lack sufficient lighting and thus was not widely received.[8,14,18] A great advance in illumination was made with Edison's electric bulb, first integrated into endoscopy by German urologist Maximillian Nitze (1848–1906). In addition to fashioning a cystoscope illuminated by a new filamentous light source, he was also the first to magnify endoscopic images with the use of lenses and develop a cystoscope capable of producing endoscopic photographs.[19–21]

At the turn of the nineteenth century, rhinology started to rapidly evolve as new techniques for visualization and access to the sinuses emerged. In 1886, Mikulicz-Radecki was the first to describe accessing the maxillary sinus through an inferior meatal antrostomy.[2] This technique was succeeded by a procedure introduced in 1893 by American George Caldwell, in which he described opening the maxillary sinus from the canine fossa and creating a rhinostomy through the inferior meatus.[22] In 1897, Henri Luc of Paris published a surgical technique identical to the one described by Caldwell, thus giving rise to the popular "Caldwell-Luc" procedure.[2,23] In 1913, Dr Mosher of Harvard University published the first description of an intranasal approach to ethmoidectomy.[24] This technique, typically performed with just a headlight, grasping forceps, and a curette, was largely abandoned due to safety concerns[25]: "...it has proved to be one of the easiest

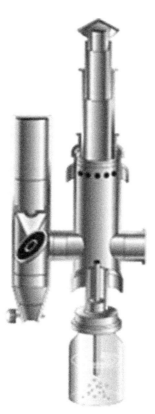

Fig. 6. Antoine Jean Desormeaux's "endoscope." (*Courtesy of* Olympus Austria, Vienna, Austria; with permission.)

operations with which to kill a patient," Mosher concluded.[26] This technique was supplanted by Lynch's external approach, which was published in 1921 and remained the preferred surgical approach to ethmoidectomy for the next 40 years.[23,27,28]

Occurring alongside these surgical advances was the gradual emergence of sinonasal endoscopy. In 1901, German otolaryngologist Hirschmann used the Nitze cystoscope, illuminated by a small electric light bulb, to examine the maxillary sinus through an enlarged tooth socket.[29,30] He also succeeded in visualizing the ethmoid sinuses after partial resection of the middle turbinate and in performing an endoscopic ethmoidectomy to clear infection.[30] Soon thereafter, Reichert performed the first endoscopic sinus surgery to treat maxillary sinus disease using a 7-mm endoscope through an oroantral fistula.[31] In 1922, Spielberg[32] published his work on visualizing the maxillary sinus with an endoscope through the inferior meatus. In 1925, Maxwell Maltz[33] introduced the "sinuscope," a device similar to the cystoscope but of smaller caliber and improved optics. He stated that akin to the importance of cytoscopes to urologists, "'sinuscopy' if practical should be an important aid to the rhinologist in his treatment of disturbances in the antrum." Despite these technical advances, they were not widely adopted and were considered by most to be technically infeasible and of little diagnostic value.[19,23] It was not until after World War II that sinonasal endoscopy started to gain traction.[30]

After a surreptitious dinner party conversation with British gastroenterologist Hugh Gainsborough, English physicist and inventor Harold Hopkins learned of the poor image quality of gastroscopy at the time. Gainsborough had implored Hopkins to improve the technology, spurring him to later develop flexible fiberoptics.[34] In 1954, Hopkins and Kapany[34] published their work in *Nature* detailing the transmission of images though flexible glass (silica) fibers. This technology was introduced previously by gynecologist Heinrich Lamm but Hopkins' fibers were a marked refinement, as they limited the high degree of light loss and image degradation associated with their previous design.[35] These new fibers were first integrated into flexible gastroscopes scopes to transmit visual information using simple light bulbs for illumination.[36] It was later realized that flexible glass fibers also could serve as light carriers and thus were later integrated into a new generation of endoscopes providing superior illumination.[29,34,36,37]

Harold Hopkins' most notable contribution, however, was the revolutionary rod-lens system in 1959 (**Fig. 7**). Rather than the conventional air interspace between glass lenses in endoscopes at the time, Hopkins placed glass rods between lenses. The rod-lens system improved image quality and brightness, allowed for a wider field of view, and permitted a smaller-diameter lens.[19,34,36,37] This great advance initially went unrecognized until Hopkins presented the idea to German equipment manufacturer Karl Storz in 1965; the rod-lens system was immediately integrated into a new generation of endoscopes that also used flexible glass fibers for bright light transmission.[36]

The unprecedented visualization and illumination provided by sinonasal endoscopy was demonstrated by the ground-breaking work of Walter Messerklinger of Austria, one of the first to use the new Storz-Hopkins endoscope. His endoscopic studies on mucociliary clearance and sinonasal anatomy led him to pioneer a number of sinonasal procedures and publish his landmark work "Endoscopy of the nose" in 1978.[3,27,29,38] Messerklinger also recognized the need for angled telescopes, as direct (0°) frontal visualization did not provide adequate visualization of the clefts of the different nasal meatuses. On request, Karl Storz constructed a variety of angled scopes (30, 70, 90, and 120°) that further enhanced one's ability to examine the nose and paranasal sinuses.[29,30]

Instruments specifically designed for endoscopic sinus surgery then gradually emerged, largely heralded by the developments of Carl Reiner of Vienna, who had

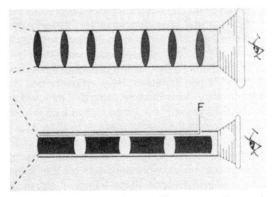

Fig. 7. Schematic of the revolutionary Hopkins rod-lens system (*bottom*) compared with the traditional endoscope containing lens interspersed with air. F, Field of view. (©2016 Photo *Courtesy of* KARL STORZ Endoscopy-America, Inc.)

the concept of designing instruments to work in parallel to the endoscope shaft. As these instruments came about, detailed endoscopic surgical technique started to develop, starting with resection of the medial infundibular wall, lateral wall of a concha bullosa, and obstructive ethmoid bulla.[30] As mucosal preservation became dogma, the need for fine, through-cutting endoscopic instrumentation was realized and created. These instruments proved to be less traumatic, safer, and allowed for more precision, particularly when addressing areas prone to sequelae from scarring, such as the frontal recess.[31]

OTHER TECHNOLOGICAL ADVANCES IN VISUALIZATION
Operating Microscope

The operating microscope, introduced by Heermann in 1958, was another important advance that provided visualization for endonasal procedures.[29,39] The microscope aided the performance of intranasal ethmoidectomy through magnification and improved illumination, but despite enhancing visualization, its use did not become popular, as it was limited by its need for a large nasal aperture maintained with a speculum and a direct line of sight of structures.[23]

Videoendoscopy

Videoendoscopy was another major technological advance, introduced by Welch Allyn Inc. in 1984 when they developed the first endoscope with a small videocamera outfitted with a CCD (charge-coupled device) sensor placed in the distal tip of the instrument replacing optical fiber image transmission.[14] Images focused on the CCD chip were converted into digital signal and processed to be displayed on a monitor.[40] Videoendoscopy has been proven to be safe and more comfortable for the surgeon compared with viewing through the endoscope directly standing or sitting over the patient.[41] Videoendoscopy also allows for instrumentation with 2 hands and by allowing procedures to be watched on a monitor, is more conducive to education and supervision.[41,42]

Improvements in viewing monitors have also changed visualization for the endoscopic surgeon. High-definition (HD) monitors allow for wider aspect ratios and improved pixel densities compared with standard definition monitors, allowing for sharper resolution, contrast, and peripheral visualization.[29] Multiple studies have demonstrated technical and diagnostic benefit of HD monitors in procedures requiring a high level of detailed visualization.[43,44] HD cameras also have improved visualization, replacing the outdated interlacing scanning system with progressive scanning, which allows for improved image resolution and elimination of image flicker.[29] Advances in digital camera chips have also improved visualization. Three-chip CCD cameras (**Fig. 8**) have replaced single-chip cameras allowing for dedicated primary color (red, blue, and green) processing rather than previous single chips outfitted with a Bayer mask that resulted in loss of color information. This has allowed for superior resolution and color fidelity.[29,45]

Xenon Light

Lighting is critical for high-quality endoscopic images. Halogen, metal halide, and xenon are the most commonly used light sources today. Light from these sources is transmitted through fiberoptic cables to provide endoscopic illumination. Xenon is typically the most preferred light source, as it provides nearly 3 times brighter light output and white light rather than yellow light, compared with its halogen predecessor. It has also been shown to last longer and produce less heat.[29]

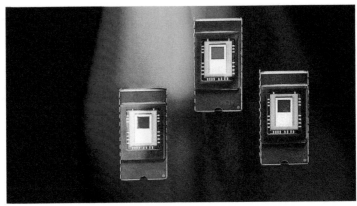

Fig. 8. Three-chip CCD video cameras offering dedicated color processing. (©2016 Photo *Courtesy of* KARL STORZ Endoscopy-America, Inc.)

Endoscopic Irrigation System

Endoscopic irrigation systems, such as the Endo-Scrub (Medtronic ENT Medtronic USA, Inc, Jacksonville, FL) deserve mention (**Fig. 9**).[46] Facilitated by a pump and sheath, a burst of irrigation cleanses the end of the endoscope allowing for maintenance of optimal visualization without removing the endoscope from the nares for manual cleaning.[47] These systems have been demonstrated to improve operative visibility in the presence of bleeding and are now routinely used in endoscopic skull base cases.[48–50]

FUTURE OF ENDOSCOPIC SINUS SURGERY
Three-Dimensional Endoscope

Stereoscopic vision refers to the ability of humans to view with both eyes, but in slightly different ways. The images from both eyes are superimposed and processed into a single image, which provides the illusion of 3-dimensional (3D) images and thus depth. Visualization during endoscopic sinus surgery is currently achieved using a 2-dimensional (2D) endoscope. However, the 2D endoscopic system does not offer the stereoscopic visualization provided by open or microscopic surgery, thus limiting the surgeon's ability to accurately gauge depth within the surgical field. To overcome the limitation of 2D visualization, the otolaryngologist must rely on anatomic knowledge and haptic cues. However, despite compensatory

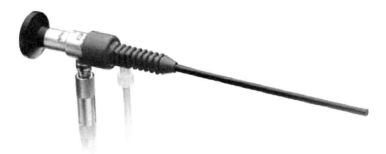

Fig. 9. Medtronic Endo-Scrub 2 lens cleaning sheath. (*Reprinted with* the permission of Medtronic, Inc. © 2016.)

mechanisms, the limitations of 2D visualization are well-recognized. A study from the general surgery literature showed that errors during laparoscopic bile duct surgery were the result of visual misperceptions rather than lack of knowledge or skill.[51]

To address this lack of stereopsis, development of 3D-visualization technology has been pursued for several decades, but has not gained traction because of technical deficiencies and because otolaryngologists have largely adapted to 2D visualization.[52,53] Stereoscopic technologies have included first-generation and second-generation dual-channel, shutter mechanism systems, time-parallel and time-multiplexed systems.[54] Recently, 3D chips were introduced and are placed on the distal end of the endoscopes to generate 3D images.[53] These various systems had several barriers to adoption, including heavy endoscopes, eyewear, and user side effects of headache and nausea. Most recently, a novel endoscope was developed which mimics an "insect eye" (**Fig. 10**). The endoscope generates multiple images by using a microscopic array of lenses positioned over a single distal-chip, thus creating stereoscopic visualization. Surgeons view the image on a stereoscopic monitor with lightweight polarized glasses.[54]

Several studies have been performed comparing the newer 3D endoscope to the standard 2D endoscope. Overall, these studies show an improvement in depth perception. Yet there is no consensus as to whether this translates to decreased surgical time or complications. Many studies report no benefit, whereas others demonstrate improved surgical efficiency.[52,55–57]

Augmented Reality Navigation System

Conventional navigation systems feature a triplanar view mode that is displayed on an additional screen from where the surgical field is viewed. Weaknesses of these systems include difficulty correlating the anatomy from the endoscopic to triplanar images and having to look away from the surgical to view the computed tomography images.[58] To address these issues, several attempts to create an augmented reality (AR) navigation system have been pursued.[59,60] AR systems fuse endoscopic images to a 3D reconstructed background, providing a stereoscopic view that is displayed on a single screen. These systems may ultimately enable safer surgery, as well as aid endoscopic surgeons in their training. Further studies must be performed to demonstrate their utility.

Robotic Endoscope Holder

Standard endoscopic sinus surgery is most commonly performed via a 2-handed technique. The otolaryngologist holds the endoscope with one hand leaving the other to manipulate instruments. When performing extended endoscopic approaches in conjunction with a neurosurgeon, a 3-handed or 4-handed technique is commonly used. In either case, 1 hand is needed to hold the endoscope and thus cannot

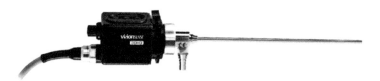

Fig. 10. Novel "insect eye" stereo-endoscope that uses an array of microscopic lenses, and single video chip to reconstruct a 3D image. (*Courtesy of* VisionSense Ltd., Philadelphia, PA; with permission.)

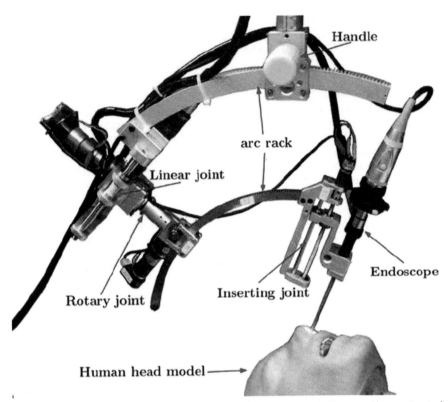

Fig. 11. Robotic arm of endoscope holder. (*From* Chan JY, Leung I, Navarro-Alarcon D, et al. Foot-controlled robotic-enabled endoscope holder (FREE) for endoscopic sinus surgery: a cadaveric feasibility study. Laryngoscope 2016;126(3):567; with permission.)

otherwise actively participate in the surgery. Furthermore, a 4-handed technique requires 2 surgeons to work within a small workspace that is not ergonomic by design. To address these issues, several attempts have been made to develop a robotic endoscope holder. None have been widely adopted because of bulky robotics and because most designs still require a separate hand to manipulate the joystick. However, recently a foot-controlled robotic-enabled endoscope holder was developed that was found to be relatively easy to use and that may reduce operative time (**Fig. 11**).[61]

REFERENCES

1. Cheever D. Anatomy eclipsed. Ann Surg 1933;98(4):792–800.
2. Nogueira JF Jr, Hermann DR, Americo Rdos R, et al. A brief history of otorhinolaryngology: otology, laryngology and rhinology. Braz J Otorhinolaryngol 2007; 73(5):693–703.
3. Kaluskar SK. Evolution of rhinology. Indian J Otolaryngol Head Neck Surg 2008; 60(2):101–5.
4. Pirsig W. History of rhinology: nasal specula around the turn of the 19th-20th century. Rhinology 1990;28(2):113–22.
5. Baber EC. Chairman's address: thirty years' progress in rhinology. Br Med J 1899;2(2015):401–2.

6. Ball JB. The progress of rhinology. West Lond Med J 1899;4:273–85.
7. Mackenzie M. Section V: the nose. In: A Manual of diseases of the throat and nose: including the pharynx, larynx, trachea, oesophagus, nose, and naso-pharynx, vol. 2. New York: William Wood and Company; 1884. p. 161–333.
8. Saxena AK. History of endoscopic surgery. In: Saxena AK, Hollwarth ME, editors. Essentials of pediatric endoscopic surgery. Berlin (Germany): Springer-Verlag Berlin Heidelberg; 2009. p. 1–15.
9. Hannan SA. The instrument that determined my practice. BMJ 2003;326:747.
10. Baber EC. Chapter IV: Examination of the nose. In: Guide to the examination of the nose. London: HK Lewis; 1886. p. 43–92.
11. Bosworth FH. Chapter I: the use of the laryngoscope. In: A manual of diseases of the throat and nose, vol. 1. New York: William Wood and Company; 1881. p. 1–32.
12. Weir N, Weir S, Stephends D. Who was who and what did they do? A biography of contributors to otolaryngology from Great Britain and Ireland. J Laryngol Otol 1987;101(1):23–87.
13. Mudry A, Holsinger C, Rameau A. Origins of the binocular head mirror: The mystery of Dr. Clar, clarified. Int J Pediatr Otorhinolaryngol 2016;80:101–5.
14. Marsh BR. Historic development of bronchoesophagology. Otolaryngol Head Neck Surg 1996;114(6):689–716.
15. Hirsch NP, Smith GB, Hirsch PO. Alfred Kirstein. Pioneer of direct laryngoscopy. Anaesthesia 1986;41(1):42–5.
16. Emani J, Baroody FM. History of nasal polyposis. In: Onerci TM, Ferguson BJ, editors. Nasal polyposis. Berlin: Springer; 2010. p. 1–7.
17. Lamaro VP. Gynaecological endoscopic surgery: past, present and future. In: O'Neill JH, editor. Sydney(Australia): St.Vincents Clinic; 2004. p. 23–9.
18. Spaner SJ, Warnock GL. A brief history of endoscopy, laparoscopy, and laparoscopic surgery. J Laparoendosc Adv Surg Tech A 1997;7(6):369–73.
19. Hoddeson EK, Wise SK, DelGaudio JM. Chapter 1: history of nasal endoscopy. In: Patel ZM, Wise SK, DelGaudio JM, editors. Office-based rhinology: principles and techniques. San Diego (CA): Plural Publishing; 2013. p. 1–4.
20. Doglietto F, Prevedello DM, Jane JA Jr, et al. Brief history of endoscopic transsphenoidal surgery—from Philipp Bozzini to the First World Congress of Endoscopic Skull Base Surgery. Neurosurg Focus 2005;19(6):E3.
21. Prevedello DM, Doglietto F, Jane JA Jr, et al. History of endoscopic skull base surgery: its evolution and current reality. J Neurosurg 2007;107(1):206–13.
22. Caldwell GW. Diseases of the accessory sinuses of the nose, and an improved method of treatment for suppuration of the maxillary antrum. NY J Med 1893; 58:526–8.
23. Leopold D. A history of rhinology in North America. Otolaryngol Head Neck Surg 1996;115(4):283–97.
24. Mosher HP. The applied anatomy and the intra-nasal surgery of the ethmoidal labyrinth. Laryngoscope 1913;23(9):881–907.
25. Lawson W. The intranasal ethmoidectomy: evolution and an assessment of the procedure. Laryngoscope 1994;104(6):1–49.
26. Mosher HP. Symposium on the ethmoid: the surgical anatomy of the ethmoidal labyrinth. Trans Am Acad Ophthalmol Otolaryngol 1929;34:376–410.
27. Kennedy DW. Sinus surgery: a century of controversy. Laryngoscope 1997; 107(1):1–5.
28. Lynch RC. The technique of a radical frontal sinus operation which has given me the best results. Laryngoscope 1921;31(1):1–5.

29. Chandra RK, Conley DB, Kern RC. Evolution of the endoscope and endoscopic sinus surgery. Otolaryngol Clin North Am 2009;42(5):747–52.

30. Messerklinger W. Background and evolution of endoscopic sinus surgery. ENT J 1994;73(7):449–50.

31. Govindaraj S, Adappa ND, Kennedy DW. Endoscopic sinus surgery: evolution and technical innovations. J Laryngol Otol 2010;124(3):242–50.

32. Spielberg W. Antroscopy of the maxillary sinus. Laryngoscope 1922;32(6):441–3.

33. Maltz M. New instrument: the sinuscope. Laryngoscope 1925;35(10):805–11.

34. Morgenstern L. Harold Hopkins (1918-1995): "There Be Light...". Surg Innov 2004;11(4):291–2.

35. Hopkins HH, Kapany NS. A flexible fiberscope, using static scanning. Nature 1954;173:39–41.

36. Linder TE, Simmen D, Stool SE. Revolutionary inventions in the 20th century, the history of endoscopy. Arch Otolaryngol Head Neck Surg 1997;123(11):1161–3.

37. Jennings CR. Harold Hopkins. Arch Otolaryngol Head Neck Surg 1998;124(9): 1042.

38. Wiedermann J, Bury SB, Singh A. Chapter 3: endoscopic diagnosis of chronic rhinosinusitis. In: Batra PS, Han JK, editors. Practical medical and surgical management of chronic rhinosinusitis. Cham (Switzerland): Springer International Publishing; 2015. p. 29–41.

39. Heermann H. Endonasal surgery with utilization of the binocular microscope. Arch Ohren Nasen Kehlkopfheilkd 1958;171(2):295–7 [in German].

40. Gross S, Kollenbrandt M. Technical evolution of medical endoscopy. Presented at Proceedings of the 13th International Student Conference on Electrical Engineering. Prague, Czech Republic; May 21, 2009. Available at: http://www.lfb.rwth-aachen.de/files/publications/2009/GRO09d.pdf. Accessed June 8, 2016.

41. Tasman AJ, Stammberger H. Video-endoscope versus endoscope for paranasal sinus surgery: influence on stereoacuity. Am J Rhinol 1998;12(6):389–92.

42. May M, Korzec KR, Mester SJ. Video telescopic sinus surgery technique for teaching. Trans Pa Acad Ophthalmol Otolaryngol 1990;42:1037–9.

43. Otto KJ, Hapner ER, Baker M, et al. Blinded evaluation of the effects of high definition and magnification on perceived image quality in laryngeal imaging. Ann Otol Rhinol Laryngol 2006;115(2):110–3.

44. Hagiike M, Phillips EH, Berci G. Performance differences in laparoscopic surgical skills between true high-definition and three-chip CCD video systems. Surg Endosc 2007;21(10):1849–54.

45. Wootton C. Chapter 6: digital image formats. In: A practical guide to video and audio compression: from sprockets and rasters to macro blocks. Burlington (MA): Focal Press; 2005. p. 115–46.

46. Shapshay SM, Rebeiz EE, Pankratov MM. Holmium:yttrium aluminum garnet laser-assisted endoscopic sinus surgery: clinical experience. Laryngoscope 1992;102(10):1177–80.

47. Stokken JK, Halderman A, Recinos PF, et al. Strategies for improving visualization during endoscopic skull base surgery. Otolaryngol Clin North Am 2016;49(1): 131–40.

48. Haruna S, Otori N, Moriyama H, et al. Endoscopic transnasal transethmosphenoidal approach for pituitary tumors: assessment of technique and postoperative findings of nasal and paranasal cavities. Auris Nasus Larynx 2007;34(1):57–63.

49. Jho H-D. Power instrumentation in endoscopic sinus surgery. Pituitary 1999;2: 139–54.

50. Kennedy DW. Functional endoscopic sinus surgery: concepts, surgical indications, and instrumentation. In: Kennedy DW, Bolger WE, Zinreich SJ, editors. Diseases of the sinuses: diagnosis and management. 1st edition. Philadelphia: PMPH USA; 2001. p. 197–210.
51. Way LW, Sterwart L, Gantert W, et al. Causes and prevention of laparoscopic bile duct injuries: analysis of 25 cases from a human factors and cognitive psychology perspective. Ann Surg 2003;237(4):460–9.
52. Tabaee A, Anand VK, Fraser JF, et al. Three dimensional endoscopic pituitary surgery neurosurgery. Neurosurgery 2009;64(5):288–93.
53. Snyderman CH, Carrau RL, Prevedello DM, et al. Technologic innovations in neuroendoscopic surgery. Otolaryngol Clin North Am 2009;42(5):883–90.
54. Singh A, Saraiya R. Three-dimensional endoscopy in sinus surgery. Curr Opin Otolaryngol Head Neck Surg 2013;21(1):3–10.
55. Brown SM, Tabaee A, Singh A, et al. Three-dimensional endoscopic sinus surgery: feasibility and technical aspects. Otolaryngol Head Neck Surg 2008; 138(3):400–2.
56. Fraser JF, Allen B, Anand VK, et al. Three-dimensional neurostereoendoscopy: subjective and objective comparison to 2D. Minim Invasive Neurosurg 2009; 52(1):25–31.
57. Kaufman Y, Sharon A, Klein O, et al. The three-dimensional "insect eye" laparoscopic imaging system: a prospective randomized study. Gynecol Surg 2007; 4(1):31s–4s.
58. Li L, Yang J, Chu Y, et al. A novel augmented reality navigation system for endoscopic sinus and skull base surgery: a feasibility study. PLoS One 2016;11(1): e0146996.
59. Caversaccio M, Garcia Giraldez J, Thoranaghatte R, et al. Augmented reality endoscopic system (ARES): preliminary results. Rhinology 2008;46(2):156–8.
60. Thoranaghatte R, Garcia J, Caversaccio M, et al. Landmark-based augmented reality system for paranasal and transnasal endoscopic surgeries. Int J Med Robot 2009;5(4):415–22.
61. Chan JY, Leung I, Navarro-Alarcon D, et al. Foot-controlled robotic-enabled endoscope holder for endoscopic sinus surgery: a cadaveric feasibility study. Laryngoscope 2016;126(3):566–9.

Organism and Microbiome Analysis

Techniques and Implications for Chronic Rhinosinusitis

Ashleigh A. Halderman, MD[a], Andrew P. Lane, MD[b],*

KEYWORDS

- Chronic rhinosinusitis • Microbiota • Metagenome • Sequence analysis, DNA
- RNA, Ribosomal, 16S

KEY POINTS

- Next-generation DNA sequencing systems are becoming increasingly accessible and affordable.
- Molecular culture-independent techniques are complementary to standard cultures and can identify a significantly greater number of bacterial organisms.
- Whole metagenome shotgun and metatranscriptomic sequencing have provided insight into complex bacterial communities and their host interactions.

INTRODUCTION

Paralleling modern advances in microbiology, our understanding of the disease process of chronic rhinosinusitis (CRS) has shifted with time as technology allows more in-depth assessments of the paranasal sinus microenvironment. Not long ago, the sinuses were thought to be sterile. The advent of culture-independent techniques has shed light onto the complex bacterial communities present in healthy paranasal sinuses, exposing limitations of standard culture in terms of the range of organisms that can be detected and grown in the laboratory setting.[1,2] Information based on morphologic characteristics of colonies grown on culture, their metabolic production or consumption, and physiologic characteristics identified by stains are all nonspecific at lower taxonomic levels.[2] With culture-dependent techniques, it is likely that microbiological results for sinonasal samples reflect in part the laboratory growth conditions rather than accurately depicting the breadth and relative abundances of resident microbes and potential pathogens. Multiple studies have shown that

[a] Department of Otolaryngology–Head and Neck Surgery, University of Southwestern Medical Center, 5303 Harry Hines Blvd, Dallas, TX 75390-9035, USA; [b] Department of Otolaryngology–Head and Neck Surgery, Johns Hopkins School of Medicine, 6th Floor, 601 North Caroline Street, Baltimore, MD 21287-0910, USA
* Corresponding author.
E-mail address: alane3@jhmi.edu

Otolaryngol Clin N Am 50 (2017) 521–532
http://dx.doi.org/10.1016/j.otc.2017.01.004
0030-6665/17/© 2017 Elsevier Inc. All rights reserved.

oto.theclinics.com

culture-independent techniques identify significantly more organisms than do standard cultures.[3–5] Furthermore, our understanding of the role of bacteria in driving CRS has begun to change as more studies have shown compelling evidence against a direct bacterial cause of the disease. This review focuses on the current technology and emerging advancements in modern microbiology.

A HISTORY OF MICROBIOLOGIC TECHNOLOGY

The microscope was known to exist as far back as the mid-1600s when Robert Hooke and later Anton van Leeuwenhoek made the first notable observations of microorganisms. However, it would not be until 200 years later when Louis Pasteur disproved the widely accepted "spontaneous generation" theory and postulated the germ theory of disease, before the field of microbiology would experience a renaissance. The 1880s proved an essential decade for techniques surrounding microbial cultivation and growth and identification that would allow the field to grow by leaps and bounds. During that 1 decade, solid media, the Petri dish, enriched culture media, plating techniques, and acid-fast and Gram stains were all invented.[6]

The late nineteenth and early twentieth centuries are sometimes referred to as "The Golden Age of Microbiology," as countless causative agents of infectious disease were identified during this time and the knowledge base grew exponentially.[6] New insights made in the 1940s and 1950s would ultimately give birth to a more modern era of microbiology and our current technology. Watson and Crick famously described the double helix structure of DNA in 1953 and the 1960s would prove a critical time for scientific advancements that would break and decipher the genetic code. A pivotal point for the field of molecular biology came in 1965, when Nobel laureate Linus Pauling introduced the concept of molecular systematics using proteins and nucleic acids to identify microorganisms.[7] The 1970s saw the development of recombinant DNA technology and the techniques to sequence DNA. Polymerase chain reaction (PCR) technology was developed in the 1980s, and the 1990s would see the achievement of the first complete genome sequence of a microorganism, *Haemophilus influenzae*. From here, we enter the modern era.

All modern methods for investigating DNA rely on the same basic steps:

1. Lyse tissue/cells
2. Isolate DNA
3. Fragment DNA
4. Sequence DNA fragments

Several methods exist for sequencing DNA. The first was described by Sanger and colleagues in the 1970s.[8,9] In this method, a single strand of DNA is divided into 4 separate sequencing reactions. Each reaction contains all 4 deoxynucleotides (dATP, dCTP, dGTP, and dTTP), DNA polymerase, and only 1 of 4 dideoxynucleotides (ddATP, ddCTP, ddGTP, or ddTTP). Starting at a specific primer, the DNA polymerase adds deoxynucleotides corresponding to the DNA template until a dideoxynucleotide is added, resulting in chain termination.[9] Originally, the fragments generated by this process were denatured into single strands and separated based on size by using gel electrophoresis. They were then visualized by autoradiography and the DNA sequence read off autoradiographs.[9] In the 1990s, the Sanger technique received updates in the form of fluorescent labeling, capillary electrophoresis, and general automation. These modifications lowered costs and improved efficiency. Yet it would be some years before DNA sequencing became feasible from a logistics, time, and expense standpoint for it to be widely accessible.

NEXT-GENERATION METHODS OF DNA SEQUENCING

Second-generation, or next-generation sequencing technologies (NGS), began to emerge throughout the mid and late 1990s and early 2000s leading to the release of the first commercially available second-generation sequencing system in 2005.[10,11] This point was critical from an accessibility standpoint, making the technology widely available at a more affordable cost for most laboratories. NGS techniques largely rely on a "sequencing-by-synthesis" design and include an initial step of DNA amplification through PCR. There are several different techniques and devices for DNA sequencing that differ in the chemistry used to determine the DNA sequence. Two techniques that exist but have not been commonly used in studies of the microbiome include Sequencing by Oligo Ligation Detection (SoLiD) (Applied Biosystems, Foster City, CA) and the Ion Personal Genome Machine (Thermo Fischer Scientific, Waltham, MA). Technologies that have been used to investigate the microbiome and even more specifically, the nasal and paranasal sinus microbiome, are discussed in greater detail as follows.

Pyrosequencing

Pyrosequencing was first described in 1998.[10] It relies on the production of light when pyrophosphate is released after nucleotide incorporation into a DNA strand. A single strand of DNA is hybridized to a primer and incubated with DNA polymerase, ATP sulfurylase, luciferase, and apyrase, as well as the substrates adenosine 5 phosphosulfate (APS) and luciferin. One at a time, the 4 nucleotides (A, C, G, and T) are added. DNA polymerase incorporates the complementary nucleotide into the DNA template and pyrophosphate is released. This is enzymatically converted to ATP, which in turn acts as a substrate for the conversion of luciferin to oxyluciferin, generating visible light that is detected by a camera and analyzed in a pyrogram. The intensity of light emitted is proportional to the number of specific nucleotides incorporated in a given area. This method was previously limited in that it could read DNA sequences of only 300 to 500 nucleotides, but this subsequently changed with commercialization of the method.

Roche (Pleasanton, CA) has developed various sequencing devices over the years that over time have increased the read lengths to up to 1000 base pairs. However, shortcomings of the platform are its high cost relative to other commercially available platforms, low throughput, low automation, and higher error rates.[12–14]

Reversible Terminator Sequencing

In the reversible terminator method, DNA is denatured into single strands and then washed with the 4 different nucleotides tagged with fluorescent dye and a reversible blocking group. One at a time, a nucleotide is incorporated. The blocking group is then cleaved, nonincorporated bases are washed away, and the next nucleotide is incorporated on rewashing with the 4 different nucleotides. The incorporation of a nucleotide results in fluorescence, with a wavelength specifically associated to that particular nucleotide and captured on imaging. This technique differs from pyrosequencing, in that each base is added one at a time, making it the more accurate of the 2 techniques.[14] Additionally, it has the greatest output of the available NGS platforms and the lowest reagent cost.[15] It does come with the disadvantages of a short read length and longer run time.[16] Sequencing devices that use this technology include the HiSeq 2000/2500 and MiSeq, both products of Illumina (San Diego, CA).

Amplicon Sequencing

Amplicon sequencing is one of the most common methods currently used for in-depth investigations into the sinonasal microbiome. Several investigators have used this technique in their recent work.[1,3,17,18] Amplicon sequencing involves amplifying and sequencing regions of highly conserved bacterial genes, which are then compared with an existing database to determine from which bacterial organisms the sequences came. These regions are also known as "markers." An ideal marker should have the following characteristics:

- It is present in every member of a population
- It differs only and always between individuals with distinct genomes
- It differs proportionally to the evolutionary distance between distinct genomes

Examples of different markers that have been used include the following:

- Ribosomal protein subunits
- Elongation factors
- RNA polymerase subunits
- cpn60 (encodes type I chaperonins)

One of the most commonly used markers is the small or 16S ribosomal RNA subunit gene, otherwise known as 16S rRNA.[19] Apart from meeting the previously listed criteria for an "ideal" maker, the 16S rRNA gene is relatively cheap and easy to sequence.[20] One or more variable regions of the 16S rRNA gene are typically used, as the entire gene is quite large at more than 1500 base pairs. In total, there are 9 different variable regions in the 16S rRNA gene. It is important to note that the use of different variable regions ultimately impacts the way operational taxonomic units (OTUs) are clustered, and thus the reported richness and evenness of a community.[21] OTUs are described in greater detail shortly. The variable regions are denoted V1, V2, V3…V9. The selection of which variable region(s) to use is based on the goals of the study. Different combinations of variable regions allow for better accuracy,[22] better estimate for species richness,[23] improved identification of specific bacterial domains,[24] and the level at which resolution (eg, species, genus) is desired.[16] An additional benefit of using the 16S rRNA gene is that the specific sequences have been determined for a vast number of bacterial species and are stored in databases, including the Ribosomal Database Project (RDP),[25] SILVA,[26] and GreenGenes.[27]

There are drawbacks to the use of 16S rRNA. Some bacteria have multiple copies of the 16S rRNA gene that can artificially increase their abundance in a sample.[28] Also, the multiple copies of the 16S rRNA within 1 bacterial genome can be highly divergent and, therefore, can be falsely identified as coming from different bacteria, which impacts reported diversity.[28] Each available marker carries its own set of advantages and disadvantages. It is essential to determine the goals of a study and the data desired before selecting a marker.

No matter what sequencing method is used, errors occur. In amplicon sequencing, horizontal transfer, incorrectly sequenced reads, and chimeric sequences (a combination of 2 or more sequences that appear as a new taxon) all can account for errors.[2,16] Various quality-based preprocessing methods have been developed to filter out low-quality reads and improve the quality of the data.[12] Additionally, tools such as UCHIME[29] and ChimeraSlayer[30] are available to identify and remove chimeric sequences.

After the processing of the data to remove errors, low-quality reads, and chimeric sequences, the sequence similarity cutoff must be determined. Typically, this is 95%, 97%, or 99%.[21] This allows for sequences that are 1% to 5% different from one another (or 95%–99% similar) to be identified as the same organism, accounting for small error reads or clonal differences within the same species. Next, the sequences are assigned to OTUs, a process referred to as "binning" or "OTU picking."

Three main approaches to binning exist. The first compares all sequences with one another without the use of outside references. Programs that perform this function include M-pick,[31] BeBAC,[32] and CROP.[33] A second method, which is taxonomy-based, uses tools such as BLAST to compare sequences with a database of known sequences to cluster OTUs.[34] A third method combines both of the these, typically starting with the taxonomy-based OTU picking and then clustering the remaining reads together based on their similarities.[35] After OTUs have been picked, the previously mentioned databases of SILVA, RDP, and GreenGenes can be used to identify which species corresponds to an OTU.

Once a sample has been separated into OTUs, the community can be analyzed by different computational methods. Parameters such as abundance, richness, and diversity both within one single population (alpha diversity) and between populations (beta diversity) can all be characterized. The data also can be represented as histograms, heat maps, and phylogenetic trees. An example of a heat map is given in **Fig. 1**. The overall process of amplicon sequencing is summarized along with whole metagenome shotgun sequencing in **Fig. 2**.

As mentioned previously, numerous investigators have used the technique of amplicon sequencing to evaluate the microbiome of the middle meatus and sinonasal cavities. The microbial composition that constitutes the microbiome of "normal sinuses" is not well defined and appears to vary quite substantially between individuals.[1,3,17,36] Some studies have demonstrated a link between species such as *Staphylococcus aureus* and *Corynebacterium tuberculostearicum* and the development of CRS.[3,37,38] Other studies have demonstrated that both diminished bacterial diversity and richness appear to be associated with the development of disease.[3,17,38]

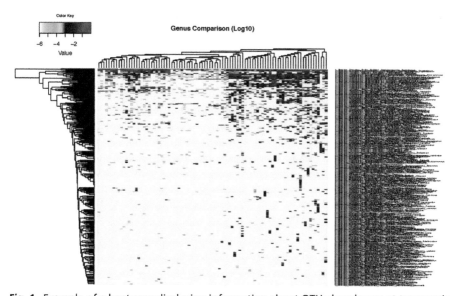

Fig. 1. Example of a heat map displaying information about OTU abundances at taxonomic levels. Various color schemes can be used to illustrate a heat map, including the commonly used rainbow map shown. A color key is included, with each color and intensity correlated with a specific value. Often added to heat maps are dendrograms, such as those at the top and left side of the figure. Dendrograms are tree diagrams that can be used to cluster both rows and columns that have similar values. It is used to cluster the genera or species (or whichever taxonomic level is being used) into groups that occur more often together.

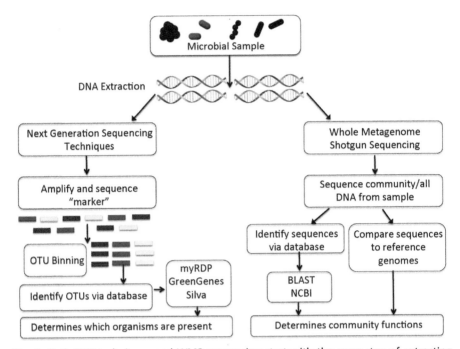

Fig. 2. Both NGS techniques and WMS sequencing start with the same step of extracting DNA from a microbial sample. Amplification of a specific marker by PCR is performed in all NGS techniques followed by sequencing the DNA. The sequences are then clustered into OTUs, and the OTUs are identified via a database to determine what organisms they came from. Alternatively, WMS sequences all DNA from a given sample instead of 1 specific marker. It does not require an amplification step. The sequences are identified either by a database, or by comparison with reference genomes. This allows for the determination of what functions a bacterial community is capable of performing.

Whole Metagenome Shotgun and Metatranscriptomic Sequencing

Whole metagenome shotgun (WMS) sequencing is the process by which all DNA (as opposed to selected portions such as 16S rRNA) from a given sample is sequenced and analyzed.[39] Initially, WMS sequencing was used on environmental samples, and in the early 2000s, led to the discovery of thousands of new viral species and determined the genomes of several bacteria and archaea that modern culture techniques had failed to isolate and grow in the laboratory.[40,41] To simplify, WMS sequencing not only determines which bacteria are present, but also which genes and gene functions are present in a community. As it does not rely on marker genes with their associated limitations stated previously, WMS sequencing is able to produce a broader or less-biased profile of a microbial community in a given sample than is amplicon sequencing.[42]

Where WMS sequences DNA, metatranscriptomic analysis sequences and analyzes RNA. It does this in a shotgun fashion by using the same technology as WMS sequencing.[43] Metatranscriptomic analysis allows one to determine which genes are being transcribed and at what level in a community. This is a relatively newer area of research, but commercially available technology and reference databases are both available at this time.[2,16] **Table 1** offers a summary and comparison of amplicon sequencing, WMS, and metatranscriptomics. The processes of WMS and

Table 1
A comparison of amplicon, whole metagenome, and metatranscriptome sequencing

Function	Amplicon Sequencing	Metagenomics	Metatranscriptomics
Sequences	Amplicon DNA	All DNA	All (m)RNA
Determines	Which bacteria are present	What the bacterial population can do	What the bacterial population is doing
Can be used to describe or calculate	Alpha diversity Beta diversity Abundance Prevalence	Differential abundance Genes Functions Pathways	Differential expression Genes Functions Pathways

metatranscriptomic sequencing have the same basic steps. Amplification via PCR is not necessary but can be included as a step as needed. Preprocessing is preformed to remove contamination (eukaryotic cells from human samples) along with quality control steps, such as the removal of redundant and low-quality sequences.[44] The next phase, if chosen, is assembly. Assembly is not required, as the preprocessed reads can be analyzed directly.[45] Assembly combines overlapping reads to form contiguous regions or "contigs" by putting together these shorter reads into longer sequences. Different assemblers are available, each of which has a unique algorithm that attempts to complete single gene sequences and, theoretically, an entire genome.[41,46] The benefit of longer sequences, and thus the reason to consider an assembly step, is improved gene-finding accuracy.[16] However, the assembly process runs the risk of creating chimeras and each assembler has its own risk to specific errors.[16] Metagenome assemblers, such as Bambus2, Genovo, and others, are available and have complicated algorithms in place to help decrease the number of chimeric contigs produced as well as algorithms to find and correct inborn errors.[47–49] Alternatively, reads can be assembled by comparing them to one of many reference databases currently available, a process called read mapping.[16] Assembly of metatranscriptomes is more difficult; however, assemblers are available, as are databases for read mapping.

Next is a step called gene finding and functional annotation. Essentially, this is the process that identifies which genes are present and their function. Gene identification can be done in 2 ways, either by predicting the presence of a gene based on certain properties of a sequence, or by comparing read sequences with a database of known protein sequences.[16] Several tools exist to carry out either of these methods. Once a gene is identified, it again must be compared with known databases of genes to determine what molecular functions or processes it does; this is known as functional annotation. By understanding what genes are present, what they do, and what their products are, an investigator can begin to understand what certain microbial communities are capable of doing. Metatranscriptomics was mentioned briefly, as it is fairly new and still in its infancy. This takes the idea of metagenomics a step further by sequencing all available RNA or mRNA from a sample to determine what a bacterial community is actually doing. Also in their infancy are metaproteomics and metametabolomics, which characterize and quantify proteins and metabolites, respectively. The ability to understand microscopic communities on this intricate of a level is an area of endless possibilities and represents a thrilling frontier.

CHRONIC RHINOSINUSITIS AND THE RELATIONSHIP WITH BACTERIA

To date, the "normal" microbiome of the paranasal sinuses has not yet been established, but wide variation among individuals has been consistently demonstrated in published studies.[1,3,17] CRS has been largely associated with decreased bacterial diversity in the paranasal sinuses and an increase in the abundance of *S aureus* and *Corynebacterium*.[3,17,36,38] Studies also have demonstrated that shifts in the microbiome occur in response to both medical therapy in the form of oral antibiotics for acute CRS exacerbations as well as topical therapies.[18,50] These findings parallel perturbations in the gut microbiota observed in response to broad-spectrum antibiotics and simple changes in diet.[51]

As mentioned previously, understanding of the role of bacteria in CRS pathogenesis is changing. It has been demonstrated that both aerobic and anaerobic bacteria can be cultured from both diseased and "healthy" control sinuses at similar rates.[52] This recognition challenges the long-held concept that the presence of pathogenic bacteria is inherently diagnostic of CRS and a primary target of medical intervention. Looking at treatment outcomes for acute rhinosinusitis, a Cochrane database review showed that regardless of treatment with placebo or an oral antibiotic, most acute rhinosinusitis cases resolved by 14 days.[53] A very slight shortened time to resolution was seen in the antibiotic group; however, 27% of patients on antibiotics experienced an adverse event compared with 15% in the placebo group.[53] The lack of a significant clinical improvement in the antibiotic treatment arm further weakens the argument that sinusitis and its associated symptoms are driven by bacteria. Further, in a randomized control trial, treatment with topical nasal steroid spray significantly improved symptoms, outperforming both an antibiotic group and a placebo group,[54] seemingly supporting the primary role of inflammation in the disease and its associated symptoms. Characteristic inflammatory profiles associated with subtypes of CRS with and without nasal polyps are now being described, with likely impact on innate antimicrobial function of the sinonasal epithelium.[55–58] Innate immune dysfunction has been implicated in the pathogenesis of CRS in general,[59–63] suggesting that host mucosal immunity underlies pathologic alterations in the sinonasal microbiota.

LOOKING TO THE FUTURE/SUMMARY

Although rapidly expanding, current understanding of the sinonasal microbiome is merely scratching the surface of the highly complex biological relationship between the host and the microbial world. Studies of the gut microbiome, which is perhaps the best understood of all anatomic subsites, have revealed intriguing associations between obesity and gut microbiome. In mice, obesity is associated with a taxonomic shift in the composition and diversity in the gut microbiota, which can be transmitted to other mice via their microbiome.[64,65] Even more fascinating are functional metagenomic studies in humans and mice that demonstrate that although obesity-associated taxonomic shifts may be inconsistent with regard to the specific taxa, the functional consistency of the shift operates similarly by enriching the capacity for energy harvest and dysregulating both fat storage and signaling within the host.[45,66] It is appealing to consider that microbiota transplants or probiotic manipulation of the paranasal sinuses may be used to reverse inflammation in CRS, or even that molecular culture-independent analyses will supplant standard culture as a clinical diagnostic tool. However, at this time, understanding of the intricate relationship between the sinus microbiome and host mucosal immunity in CRS remains nascent. As such, the utility of the technologies outlined in this review remains largely within the research arena, rather than in patient care. With their continued use and refinement, greater insight into the role of sinonasal microbes in health and in CRS pathogenesis will likely emerge, prompting identification of relevant biomarkers and the development of novel therapeutic interventions for CRS.

REFERENCES

1. Ramakrishnan VR, Feazel LM, Gitomer SA, et al. The microbiome of the middle meatus in healthy adults. PLoS One 2013;8(12):e85507.

2. Morgan XC, Huttenhower C. Chapter 12: Human microbiome analysis. PLoS Comput Biol 2012;8(12):e1002808.

3. Feazel LM, Robertson CE, Ramakrishnan VR, et al. Microbiome complexity and *Staphylococcus aureus* in chronic rhinosinusitis. Laryngoscope 2012;122(2): 467–72.

4. Hauser LJ, Feazel LM, Ir D, et al. Sinus culture poorly predicts resident microbiota. Int Forum Allergy Rhinol 2015;5(1):3–9.

5. Stephenson MF, Mfuna L, Dowd SE, et al. Molecular characterization of the polymicrobial flora in chronic rhinosinusitis. J Otolaryngol Head Neck Surg 2010; 39(2):182–7.

6. Significant Events in Microbiology 1861-1999. American Society for Microbiology. 2015. Available at: www.asm.org/index.php/choma3. Accessed July 15, 2016.

7. Zuckerkandl E, Pauling L. Molecules as documents of evolutionary history. J Theor Biol 1965;8(2):357–66.

8. Sanger F, Coulson AR. A rapid method for determining sequences in DNA by primed synthesis with DNA polymerase. J Mol Biol 1975;94(3):441–8.

9. Sanger F, Nicklen S, Coulson AR. DNA sequencing with chain-terminating inhibitors. Proc Natl Acad Sci U S A 1977;74(12):5463–7.

10. Ronaghi M, Uhlen M, Nyren P. A sequencing method based on real-time pyrophosphate. Science 1998;281(5375):363, 365.

11. Metzker ML. Emerging technologies in DNA sequencing. Genome Res 2005; 15(12):1767–76.

12. Huse SM, Huber JA, Morrison HG, et al. Accuracy and quality of massively parallel DNA pyrosequencing. Genome Biol 2007;8(7):R143.

13. Gilles A, Meglecz E, Pech N, et al. Accuracy and quality assessment of 454 GS-FLX Titanium pyrosequencing. BMC Genomics 2011;12:245.

14. Luo C, Tsementzi D, Kyrpides N, et al. Direct comparisons of Illumina vs. Roche 454 sequencing technologies on the same microbial community DNA sample. PLoS One 2012;7(2):e30087.

15. Liu L, Li Y, Li S, et al. Comparison of next-generation sequencing systems. J Biomed Biotechnol 2012;2012:251364.

16. Di Bella JM, Bao Y, Gloor GB, et al. High throughput sequencing methods and analysis for microbiome research. J Microbiol Methods 2013;95(3):401–14.

17. Biswas K, Hoggard M, Jain R, et al. The nasal microbiota in health and disease: variation within and between subjects. Front Microbiol 2015;9:134.

18. Liu CM, Kohanski MA, Mendiola M, et al. Impact of saline irrigation and topical corticosteroids on the postsurgical sinonasal microbiota. Int Forum Allergy Rhinol 2015;5(3):185–90.

19. Tringe SG, Hugenholtz P. A renaissance for the pioneering 16S rRNA gene. Curr Opin Microbiol 2008;11(5):442–6.

20. Caporaso JG, Kuczynski J, Stombaugh J, et al. QIIME allows analysis of high-throughput community sequencing data. Nat Methods 2010;7(5):335–6.

21. Schloss PD. The effects of alignment quality, distance calculation method, sequence filtering, and region on the analysis of 16S rRNA gene-based studies. PLoS Comput Biol 2010;6(7):e1000844.

22. Liu Z, DeSantis TZ, Andersen GL, et al. Accurate taxonomy assignments from 16S rRNA sequences produced by highly parallel pyrosequencers. Nucleic Acids Res 2008;36(18):e120.
23. Youssef N, Sheik CS, Krumholz LR, et al. Comparison of species richness estimates obtained using nearly complete fragments and simulated pyrosequencing-generated fragments in 16S rRNA gene-based environmental surveys. Appl Environ Microbiol 2009;75(16):5227–36.
24. Gilbert JA, Meyer F, Antonopoulos D, et al. Meeting report: the terabase metagenomics workshop and the vision of an Earth microbiome project. Stand Genomic Sci 2010;3(3):243–8.
25. Cole JR, Wang Q, Cardenas E, et al. The Ribosomal Database Project: improved alignments and new tools for rRNA analysis. Nucleic Acids Res 2009; 37(Database issue):D141–5.
26. Pruesse E, Quast C, Knittel K, et al. SILVA: a comprehensive online resource for quality checked and aligned ribosomal RNA sequence data compatible with ARB. Nucleic Acids Res 2007;35(21):7188–96.
27. DeSantis TZ, Hugenholtz P, Larsen N, et al. Greengenes, a chimera-checked 16S rRNA gene database and workbench compatible with ARB. Appl Environ Microbiol 2006;72(7):5069–72.
28. Acinas SG, Marcelino LA, Klepac-Ceraj V, et al. Divergence and redundancy of 16S rRNA sequences in genomes with multiple rrn operons. J Bacteriol 2004; 186(9):2629–35.
29. Edgar RC, Haas BJ, Clemente JC, et al. UCHIME improves sensitivity and speed of chimera detection. Bioinformatics 2011;27(16):2194–200.
30. Haas BJ, Gevers D, Earl AM, et al. Chimeric 16S rRNA sequence formation and detection in Sanger and 454-pyrosequenced PCR amplicons. Genome Res 2011; 21(3):494–504.
31. Wang X, Yao J, Sun Y, et al. M-pick, a modularity-based method for OTU picking of 16S rRNA sequences. BMC Bioinformatics 2013;14:43.
32. Cheng L, Walker AW, Corander J. Bayesian estimation of bacterial community composition from 454 sequencing data. Nucleic Acids Res 2012;40(12):5240–9.
33. Hao X, Jiang R, Chen T. Clustering 16S rRNA for OTU prediction: a method of unsupervised Bayesian clustering. Bioinformatics 2011;27(5):611–8.
34. Altschul SF, Madden TL, Schaffer AA, et al. Gapped BLAST and PSI-BLAST: a new generation of protein database search programs. Nucleic Acids Res 1997; 25(17):3389–402.
35. Bik HM, Porazinska DL, Creer S, et al. Sequencing our way towards understanding global eukaryotic biodiversity. Trends Ecol Evol 2012;27(4):233–43.
36. Boase S, Foreman A, Cleland E, et al. The microbiome of chronic rhinosinusitis: culture, molecular diagnostics and biofilm detection. BMC Infect Dis 2013;13: 210.
37. Ramakrishnan VR, Feazel LM, Abrass LJ, et al. Prevalence and abundance of Staphylococcus aureus in the middle meatus of patients with chronic rhinosinusitis, nasal polyps, and asthma. Int Forum Allergy Rhinol 2013;3(4):267–71.
38. Abreu NA, Nagalingam NA, Song Y, et al. Sinus microbiome diversity depletion and Corynebacterium tuberculostearicum enrichment mediates rhinosinusitis. Sci Transl Med 2012;4(151):151ra124.
39. Riesenfeld CS, Schloss PD, Handelsman J. Metagenomics: genomic analysis of microbial communities. Annu Rev Genet 2004;38:525–52.
40. Breitbart M, Salamon P, Andresen B, et al. Genomic analysis of uncultured marine viral communities. Proc Natl Acad Sci U S A 2002;99(22):14250–5.

41. Tyson GW, Chapman J, Hugenholtz P, et al. Community structure and metabolism through reconstruction of microbial genomes from the environment. Nature 2004; 428(6978):37–43.

42. Sogin ML, Morrison HG, Huber JA, et al. Microbial diversity in the deep sea and the underexplored "rare biosphere. Proc Natl Acad Sci U S A 2006;103(32): 12115–20.

43. Gilbert JA, Field D, Huang Y, et al. Detection of large numbers of novel sequences in the metatranscriptomes of complex marine microbial communities. PLoS One 2008;3(8):e3042.

44. Mende DR, Waller AS, Sunagawa S, et al. Assessment of metagenomic assembly using simulated next generation sequencing data. PLoS One 2012;7(2):e31386.

45. Turnbaugh PJ, Hamady M, Yatsunenko T, et al. A core gut microbiome in obese and lean twins. Nature 2009;457(7228):480–4.

46. Hoff KJ, Lingner T, Meinicke P, et al. Orphelia: predicting genes in metagenomic sequencing reads. Nucleic Acids Res 2009;37(Web Server issue):W101–5.

47. Koren S, Treangen TJ, Pop M. Bambus 2: scaffolding metagenomes. Bioinformatics 2011;27(21):2964–71.

48. Laserson J, Jojic V, Koller D. Genovo: de novo assembly for metagenomes. J Comput Biol 2011;18(3):429–43.

49. Kelley DR, Liu B, Delcher AL, et al. Gene prediction with Glimmer for metagenomic sequences augmented by classification and clustering. Nucleic Acids Res 2012;40(1):e9.

50. Liu CM, Soldanova K, Nordstrom L, et al. Medical therapy reduces microbiota diversity and evenness in surgically recalcitrant chronic rhinosinusitis. Int Forum Allergy Rhinol 2013;3(10):775–81.

51. Dethlefsen L, Relman DA. Incomplete recovery and individualized responses of the human distal gut microbiota to repeated antibiotic perturbation. Proc Natl Acad Sci U S A 2011;108(Suppl 1):4554–61.

52. Bhattacharyya N. Bacterial infection in chronic rhinosinusitis: a controlled paired analysis. Am J Rhinol 2005;19(6):544–8.

53. Lemiengre MB, van Driel ML, Merenstein D, et al. Antibiotics for clinically diagnosed acute rhinosinusitis in adults. Cochrane Database Syst Rev 2012;(10):CD006089.

54. Meltzer EO, Bachert C, Staudinger H. Treating acute rhinosinusitis: comparing efficacy and safety of mometasone furoate nasal spray, amoxicillin, and placebo. J Allergy Clin Immunol 2005;116(6):1289–95.

55. Van Zele T, Claeys S, Gevaert P, et al. Differentiation of chronic sinus diseases by measurement of inflammatory mediators. Allergy 2006;61(11):1280–9.

56. Zhang N, Van Zele T, Perez-Novo C, et al. Different types of T-effector cells orchestrate mucosal inflammation in chronic sinus disease. J Allergy Clin Immunol 2008;122(5):961–8.

57. Jyonouchi H, Sun S, Le H, et al. Evidence of dysregulated cytokine production by sinus lavage and peripheral blood mononuclear cells in patients with treatment-resistant chronic rhinosinusitis. Arch Otolaryngol Head Neck Surg 2001;127(12): 1488–94.

58. Ramanathan M Jr, Lee WK, Spannhake EW, et al. Th2 cytokines associated with chronic rhinosinusitis with polyps down-regulate the antimicrobial immune function of human sinonasal epithelial cells. Am J Rhinol 2008;22(2):115–21.

59. Woods CM, Lee VS, Hussey DJ, et al. Lysozyme expression is increased in the sinus mucosa of patients with chronic rhinosinusitis. Rhinology 2012;50(2): 147–56.

60. Cui YH, Zhang F, Xiong ZG, et al. Increased serum complement component 3 and mannose-binding lectin levels in adult Chinese patients with chronic rhinosinusitis. Rhinology 2009;47(2):187–91.

61. Ramanathan M Jr, Lee WK, Dubin MG, et al. Sinonasal epithelial cell expression of toll-like receptor 9 is decreased in chronic rhinosinusitis with polyps. Am J Rhinol 2007;21(1):110–6.

62. Lane AP, Truong-Tran QA, Schleimer RP. Altered expression of genes associated with innate immunity and inflammation in recalcitrant rhinosinusitis with polyps. Am J Rhinol 2006;20(2):138–44.

63. Lee RJ, Kofonow JM, Rosen PL, et al. Bitter and sweet taste receptors regulate human upper respiratory innate immunity. J Clin Invest 2014;124(3):1393–405.

64. Ley RE, Backhed F, Turnbaugh P, et al. Obesity alters gut microbial ecology. Proc Natl Acad Sci U S A 2005;102(31):11070–5.

65. Turnbaugh PJ, Ley RE, Mahowald MA, et al. An obesity-associated gut microbiome with increased capacity for energy harvest. Nature 2006;444(7122):1027–31.

66. Turnbaugh PJ, Backhed F, Fulton L, et al. Diet-induced obesity is linked to marked but reversible alterations in the mouse distal gut microbiome. Cell Host Microbe 2008;3(4):213–23.

Topical Drug Therapies for Chronic Rhinosinusitis

Lauren J. Luk, MD, John M. DelGaudio, MD*

KEYWORDS

- Sinus irrigations • Nebulizers • Topical • Chronic rhinosinusitis • Steroids

KEY POINTS

- Chronic rhinosinusitis (CRS) is an inflammatory syndrome involving the nose and paranasal sinuses of multifactorial etiology that results in common signs and symptoms.
- Medical treatment has shifted toward addressing inflammation, with topical saline and corticosteroids used in previously operated patients, reserving topical antibiotics for culture-directed acute exacerbations.
- Topical therapies discussed in this article include saline, corticosteroids, antibiotics, and antifungals.

SALINE IRRIGATION

Nasal irrigation remains one of the oldest and most effective topical therapies for chronic rhinosinusitis (CRS). The ancient Hindu practice of *Ayurveda* provides the earliest record of nasal irrigation.[1] It was customary to perform the *jala-neti* as part of *soucha* (personal hygiene according to the scriptures). By purifying the nose, a higher state of meditation could be achieved because clear breathing led to clear thinking. The simplest method of nasal cleansing was to sniff water from cupped hands and blow it out, which is also a step in Muslim ablutions practice. *Neti* is the Sanskrit word for nasal cleaning, and the design of today's genie-lamp shaped "netipot" is largely unchanged over centuries.

Many saline delivery devices have been proposed, including low-flow devices such as the aerosol spray bottle and nebulizer, and high-flow devices such as the bulb syringe, squeeze bottle, and dental pulse irrigator. Studies have shown that high-volume devices with delivery of greater than 100 mL of saline are superior to low-volume sprays. A study by Pynnonen and colleagues randomized 127 patients with acute rhinosinusitis/CRS and 4 weeks of nasal symptoms to treatment with either large-volume irrigation or low-volume spray delivery of isotonic saline.[2] They found that large-volume irrigation

Disclosure Statement: Dr. DelGaudio receives grant support from Spirox.
Department of Otolaryngology–Head and Neck Surgery, Emory University, Emory University, Medical Office Tower, 550 Peachtree Street Northeast, Suite 1135, Atlanta, GA 30308, USA
* Corresponding author.
E-mail address: jdelgau@emory.edu

Otolaryngol Clin N Am 50 (2017) 533–543
http://dx.doi.org/10.1016/j.otc.2017.01.005
oto.theclinics.com

significantly improved Sino-Nasal Outcome Test (SNOT) scores at 2, 4, and 8 weeks as compared with spray.[2] In addition, there is poor distribution of saline throughout the sinuses with the low-volume spray, even after sinus surgery.[2]

There has also been debate regarding the most effective formulation of saline. A randomized controlled trial by Hauptman and Ryan demonstrated that both isotonic and hypertonic saline improved saccharine clearance time.[3] However, hypertonic saline was associated with increased nasal irritation as well as a lack of improvement in nasal patency as reported by patients.[3] The authors hypothesized that hypertonic saline may induce neural responses that lead to localized vasodilation resulting in local swelling and obstruction.[3] However, other studies have concluded that both formulations are equally effective.[4]

Saline irrigation has many benefits, including removing environmental allergens, clearing excess mucus, and improving mucociliary clearance.[5,6] Indications for use in CRS include adjunctive medical treatment with corticosteroids as well as postoperative therapy. A 2009 Cochrane review, which included 8 randomized, controlled trials, concluded that the "beneficial effects of topical saline outweigh minor side effects."[4,5] Pooled data from 3 randomized, controlled trials demonstrated that use of topical saline was associated with statistically significant improvement in symptom scores and disease specific quality of life as compared with no treatment.[4,5] However, these data included heterogeneous studies of patients with allergic rhinitis, CRS, recurrent acute sinusitis, and many who had undergone prior sinus surgery, treated with hypertonic and isotonic saline delivered by both irrigation and spray. In 2011, Wei and colleagues[6] reviewed 16 randomized, controlled trials and concluded that saline is beneficial in treating CRS as a sole modality as well as treatment adjunct after surgery. However, patients experienced less improvement of symptoms when treated with saline alone when directly compared with topical corticosteroid therapy.[7]

Topical saline irrigation is also useful in the postoperative period in terms of patient symptoms as well as early endoscopic appearance of the sinuses.[8] Patients with mild to moderate CRS (Lund-Mackay < or =12) demonstrate significant symptomatic improvement with postoperative debridement with adjunctive saline versus debridement alone.[9] However, patients with more severe disease did not demonstrate statistically significant benefits.

Although use of topical saline is generally well-tolerated, side effects including nasal irritation/burning, sore throat, otalgia or aural fullness, epistaxis, postnasal drainage, and headache have been reported.[8] Bacterial colonization of irrigation devices has been established but the impact on CRS disease course is unclear.[9,10] The presence of bacteria cultured from irrigation bottles has not been associated with increased rates of postoperative infections.[10,11] However, physicians should encourage patients to clean their nasal irrigation devices regularly to minimize them as potential infection sources. In addition, limited studies suggest no effect of high-volume saline irrigation on sinus microbiota (with or without budesonide) as opposed to topical intranasal steroid application.[12] Although extremely rare, primary amebic meningoencephalitis deaths associated with sinus irrigations with contaminated water have been reported in the literature.[13]

In summary, saline nasal irrigations are a beneficial adjunctive therapy with minimal side effects for patients with CRS as supported by multiple randomized, controlled trials.

TOPICAL CORTICOSTEROIDS

Topical corticosteroids, initially developed for the long-term management of lower airway disease, are now a mainstay of CRS therapy. Beclomethasone dipropionate was the first clinically active aerosolized corticosteroid discovered in 1972.[14] It was found to have increased potency with fewer systemic side effects as compared with oral hydrocortisone or dexamethasone, which led to improved patient compliance. Major adverse effects from oral corticosteroids are related to suppression of the hypothalamic–pituitary–adrenal (HPA) axis function and the development of iatrogenic Cushing's syndrome (cardiovascular disease, thromboembolic events, weight gain, glucose intolerance, osteoporosis/avascular necrosis of bone, obesity, skin changes, neuropsychological changes, immune deficiency, cataracts, serous chorioretinopathy, and increased intraocular pressure).[15] Other topical steroid sprays were developed including mometasone furoate and fluticasone proprionate. Topical steroid drops, including dexamethasone and methylprednisolone, have been used off-label to treat refractory cases of CRS as well.[16] Most recently, budesonide has been borrowed from the pulmonary literature and used in an atomizer or drop formulation or in large-volume irrigations to treat CRS.[17]

Corticosteroids have multiple mechanisms of action in suppressing inflammation in CRS. Chiefly, they reverse histone acetylation of activated inflammatory genes in the nucleus to decrease production of cytokines, chemokines, adhesion molecules, inflammatory enzymes, and receptors.[18] They promote transcription of antiinflammatory proteins such as mitogen activated kinase phosphatase-1.[19] They inhibit macrophage presentation of antigens to lymphocytes thus reducing lymphocyte activation, differentiation, and cytokine release. Ultimately, they reduce mucosal inflammation, decrease vascular permeability, and reduce glycoprotein release.[7]

Topical corticosteroids use for CRS with (CRSwNP) and without nasal polyposis (CRSsNP) is well-supported in the literature. In 2008, Joe and colleagues[20] performed a metaanalysis of 6 randomized, controlled trials (all double-blinded with placebo control) of CRSwNP treated with either mometasone or budesonide and demonstrated significant decrease in polyp size. In addition, decrease in polyp size directly correlated with decrease in symptom score.[7] Although improvement in symptoms such as nasal congestion and rhinorrhea after treatment with topical steroids is well-established, improvement in smell is more controversial. Out of 22 published studies, 14 reported improved subjective olfactory scores, whereas only 1 of 6 published studies demonstrated an objective improvement in olfactory score after treatment with topical steroids alone.[21]

Recently, topical corticosteroids have also been shown to be beneficial in treating CRSsNP. In 2009, a metaanalysis including 5 randomized, controlled trials performed by Kalish and colleagues[22] concluded there was insufficient evidence to demonstrate overall benefit of topical steroids despite low side effect profile. In 2011, Snidvongs and colleagues[23] published a Cochrane metaanalysis of 10 randomized, controlled trials (590 patients) and concluded that the benefits of topical steroids treatment for CRSsNP outweighed the minor adverse effects. Compared with placebo, topical steroids significantly improved symptom scores. The most commonly reported adverse side effects included epistaxis and headache.

The newest Cochrane review published in 2016 by Chong and colleagues[24] combined 18 randomized, controlled trials including 2738 patients; 14 randomized, controlled trials investigated CRSwNP patients and 4 randomized, controlled trials studied CRSsNP patients. The authors concluded that there was very little information about quality of life (very low-quality evidence), although there seems to be improvement in disease severity for all symptoms (low-quality evidence). There was a moderate sized benefit specifically for nasal blockage and a small benefit for rhinorrhea (moderate quality evidence). Many studies mentioned the risk of local irritation but did not quantify this risk (low-quality evidence). The risk of epistaxis was increased (high-quality evidence), but the clinical relevance is unclear because the studies included all levels of severity. Another Cochrane review by this group concluded that there was insufficient evidence to recommend 1 type of intranasal steroid over another.[25] In addition, no conclusions could be drawn about the relative effectiveness of the corticosteroid formulations (spray vs aerosol).

Systemic steroids are often indicated postoperatively, especially in cases of severe inflammation with polyposis in conjunction with topical corticosteroid sprays, which are usually started 1 week after surgery.[26] Numerous steroid preparations have been described in the literature including beclomethasone dipropionate,[27] prednisolone acetate,[28] mometasone furoate,[29] triamcinolone acetonide,[25] fluticasone propnionate[30] among others (**Table 1**). However, the optimal topical steroid preparation and delivery have not been established.[25]

Recent studies suggest that off-label use of budesonide respules may offer superior postoperative symptom control as compared with traditional nasal sprays. Budesonide is most commonly used in a high-volume irrigation (0.5–1.0 mg of budesonide in 240 mL of normal saline), which provides a higher concentration of steroid than traditional nasal sprays. Cadaver studies have shown improved distribution of dye

Table 1
Topical steroid preparations

Name	Dose (per Spray)	Frequency	Notes
Beclomethasone dipropionate	40 or 80 μg	1 spray per nostril bid	
Budesonide spray	32 μg	1–4 sprays per nostril once daily	For CRSwNP – 128 μg (2 sprays per nostril) once daily
Budesonide respules	0.5–1 mg	1. Direct drops (1 mL in each nostril bid) 2. High-volume irrigation bid 3. Mucosal atomizer device, 1 mL (0.25 mg) in each nostril bid	For irrigation, dissolve 1 mg in 240 mL of normal saline and irrigate 60 mL per nostril bid
Ciclesonide	50 μg	2 sprays per nostril once daily	
Ciprofloxacin/ dexamethasone otic drops Prednisolone acetate ophthalmic drops	3 mg/mL ciprofloxacin 1 mg/mL dexamethasone 1 mg/mL prednisolone	2 drops bid per nostril twice daily	Can be tapered to once daily and then every other day
Flunisolide	25 μg	2 sprays per nostril tid	
Fluticasone propionate	50 μg	2 sprays per nostril bid	
Fluticasone furoate	27.5 μg	2 sprays per nostril once daily	May decrease to 1 spray per nostril once daily after symptoms controlled
Mometasone furoate	50 μg	1 spray per nostril bid	
Triamcinolone acetonide	55 μg	1–2 sprays per nostril once daily	

with high-volume sprays as compared with nasal sprays. A randomized, controlled trial of 30 CRSwNP patients demonstrates the most improved postoperative SNOT scores in patients treated with budesonide delivered by mucosal atomizer followed by budesonide vertex to floor respules, and both treatments were superior to fluticasone.[31] The mucosal atomization device has been proposed recently as an alternative delivery method of budesonide. A small study of CRSsNP patients randomized to budesonide delivered by mucosal atomization device demonstrated greater SNOT improvement as compared with those treated with budesonide via high-volume irrigation.[17,31] In addition, a cadaver study demonstrates superior distribution of fluorescein dye via mucosal atomization device using the Mygind[32] (lying with the head back) versus the Moffett[33] (head down and forward) head position.[34]

The development of topical nasal steroids has also helped to advance endoscopic sinus surgery, especially in the case of refractory frontal sinus disease. Frontal ostium restenosis of up to 60% within the first year after frontal sinus drillout (modified Lothrop) is a well-described complication of surgery.[35–37] Poor outcomes led many to abandon the procedure.[36] Off-label use of topical steroid drops including dexamethasone, methylprednisone, and ciprodex (2 drops to affected area twice daily followed by taper to once daily and then every other day for maintenance after surgery) has been described to help prevent ostia stenosis and is regarded to be generally safe (see **Table 1**).[16,38] However, in a retrospective study of 36 patients, 1 patient discontinued therapy owing to suppressed morning cortisol levels within 2 months of treatment.[16] However, the advent of topical budesonide along with improved equipment for drilling and visualization has improved the success and popularity of the modified Lothrop procedure for refractory frontal disease.[36,39]

Although intranasal topical corticosteroids are generally safe, they are not without local and systemic side effects. Mild epistaxis associated with topical steroid use may be the result of incorrect usage (aiming toward the septum instead of aiming toward the outer corner of the eye) and the steroid's intrinsic vasoconstrictor activity.[40] Several factors including corticosteroid formulation, dose, delivery mode, and severity of disease contribute to systemic absorption and adverse effects. The bioavailability of fluticasone and mometasone is estimated to be at 1%, whereas the budesonide and triamcinolone may be closer to 40% to 50%.[41] Extensive prospective studies of low bioavailability intranasal steroids administered at typical doses have not demonstrated any clinically significant HPA axis suppression.[40] The authors recommend using a low bioavailability intranasal steroid, especially if the patient has concomitant asthma and is being treated with an inhaled steroid as well.

The safety profile of budesonide is currently being investigated with regard to intraocular pressure and HPA axis suppression. In small prospective studies, budesonide irrigations do not seem to affect intraocular pressure within a 1-month[42] to 22-month period.[43] Subclinical HPA axis suppression with prolonged use of budesonide has been described in the literature. A prospective study of 48 patients by Soudry and colleagues[43] recently reported low stimulated cortisol levels in 23% of the patients after at least 6 months of treatment with topical budesonide (mean use, 22 months). All patients were asymptomatic and were able to continue budesonide irrigation with supervision of an endocrinologist. As expected, there was a significant correlation between concurrent inhaled and intranasal steroid use and low stimulated cortisol levels. A prior study by Smith and colleagues[36] did not demonstrate HPA axis suppression with a similar duration of budesonide use despite concurrent use of intranasal budesonide and inhaled steroids for asthma in 62% of patients. Thus, the prevalence and significance of HPA axis suppression in patients using concurrent oral or inhaled steroids with topical budesonide is currently unknown.

No specific studies have been performed on pregnant patients with CRS. However, adverse outcomes of topical steroid use can be extrapolated from studies of pregnant patients with asthma or rhinitis. The US Food and Drug Administration has classified intranasal steroids as category C with the exception of budesonide, which is category B in early pregnancy.[44] A large randomized, controlled trial demonstrated no difference in adverse outcomes of pregnancy in pregnant patients treated with inhaled budesonide versus placebo.[44] A randomized, controlled trial of 27 patients diagnosed with pregnancy rhinitis treated with fluticasone propionate for 8 weeks after the first trimester demonstrates no significant effects on morning and evening cortisol levels, on ultrasound measures of fetal growth, or on pregnancy outcomes.[45] However, treatment with fluticasone also did not improve objective nasal obstruction significantly as measured by acoustic rhinometry and subjective symptom scores. Inhaled beclomethasone and triamcinolone are not associated with preeclampsia, preterm weight, or low birth weight in pregnant asthmatic women.[41] Pregnant patients should be counseled properly regarding adverse effects of topical steroid use despite limited evidence demonstrating its safety.

In summary, topical corticosteroids are beneficial in treatment of CRS with and without nasal polyposis as supported but multiple randomized controlled trials. Optimal drug, dosage, and delivery to balance therapeutic benefits with adverse effects have yet to be determined.

TOPICAL ANTIBIOTICS

Topical and oral antibiotics were once the cornerstone of CRS medical therapy because the inflammation seen in CRS was postulated to be a result of a bacterial sinus infection. Bacterial biofilms decrease the oxygen concentration and core pH in the sinuses, allowing bacteria to downregulate metabolic activity with subsequent antibiotic resistance.[46] However, over time there has been a paradigm shift away from an infectious etiology of CRS toward a more generalized inflammatory etiology. Initial retrospective studies demonstrated that treatment with topical steroids led to improvement in facial pain and purulent rhinorrhea.[47] However, subsequent randomized, controlled trials and metaanalyses have not demonstrated the same benefit in symptoms or sinus-specific quality of life.[6,7,48] Topical antibiotic therapy should be aimed toward treating acute exacerbations of CRS.

Topical antibiotics may play a role in treating methicillin-resistant *Staphylococcus aureus*–positive CRS exacerbations (**Table 2**). Mupirocin inhibits RNA and protein synthesis. Topical mupirocin used either as an ointment or as a rinse is 90% effective in eradicating methicillin-resistant *S aureus* colonization within 5 days.[49] However, the durability of its effectiveness is controversial with an eradication rate of 60% at longer follow-up.[49] Topical mupirocin is also effective against staph aureus biofilms as compared with oral ciprofloxacin and vancomycin.[50]

Aerosolized topical tobramycin has also been shown to achieve 10 times the minimum inhibitory concentration against most pseudomonas isolates while maintaining low serum concentration.[51] In addition, use of aerosolized tobramycin after endoscopic sinus surgery in patients with cystic fibrosis and CRS significantly decreases the rate of revision surgery.[52]

Adverse effects of topical antibiotics are similar to other topical therapies, including postnasal drainage, nasal irritation, dryness, burning, itching, otalgia, and sore throat. In summary, randomized, controlled trials do not support the widespread, routine use of topical antibiotics in CRS. They may be used judiciously in a culture-directed fashion in patients who do not respond to medical and surgical management.

Table 2
Topical antibiotic and antifungal therapy

Drug	Dosage	Activity	Notes
Gentamicin	95 mg every 12 h nebulized or 80 mg mixed in 500 mL of normal saline; irrigate each nostril with up to 60 mL × 3 wk	Gram-negative organisms including *Escherichia coli*	
Mupirocin	Topical ointment or as suspension (5 g ointment in 45 mL of normal saline, irrigate each nostril with 10 mL bid) for 5 d	*Staphylococcus aureus* and *S pyogenes*	Treatment may need to be repeated over time
Tobramycin	95 mg every 12 h nebulized × 3 wk	Gram-negative organisms including *Pseudomonas*	Well-tolerated by patients with cystic fibrosis
Amphotericin B topical	100 μg/mL; 20 mL bid per nostril as adjunct to intravenous therapy in invasive fungal sinusitis	Most fungi including *Mucoraecea* and most *Aspergillus*	Variable resistant: *Aspergillus and Zygomycetes* Resistant: *Psudollescheria boydii* and *Fusarium*

TOPICAL ANTIFUNGALS

In the late 1990s, novel techniques of collecting and culturing nasal secretions led to the discovery of positive fungal cultures and eosinophilic mucin in 96% of patients with CRS.[53] It was postulated that fungal elements became trapped in the sinonasal mucus and triggered an immune reaction, leading to recruitment of eosinophils that attacked the fungi and released inflammatory toxic mediators, resulting in CRS.[54] However, fungal cultures were positive in 100% of control subjects.[53] Topical antifungal therapy was developed to eradicate this potential source of infection and inflammation. Several observational studies demonstrated improvement of subjective symptoms and resolution of nasal polyposis after treatment with topical amphotericin B nasal lavage.[55,56] However, these studies were subject to observer bias and did not have an adequate control group. After the failure of multiple randomized, controlled trials[57,58] and metaanalyses[59,60] to show symptomatic benefit with topical antifungal therapy compared with placebo, fungi are now recognized as physiologic flora of the upper respiratory tract and "innocent bystanders" in the vast majority of patients with CRS.[54] In a subset of patients with CRS identified with allergic fungal sinusitis, fungal elements play a greater role in inflammation.[53]

Amphotericin B binds ergosterol in the fungal cell membrane and creates a transmembrane channel resulting in fungal death. Amphotericin B covers most fungi but there may be resistant strains of *Aspergillis* and *Zygomycetes*. *Pseudollescheria boydii* and *Fusarium* are resistant. The topical preparation attempts to limit side effects such as nephrotoxicity seen in the intravenous preparation. Adverse drug effects include local irritation (nasal burning, dryness, bleeding, itching), muscle aches, facial pain, nasal congestion, rhinorrhea, and respiratory symptoms (asthma attack, bronchitis, cough).[54]

Currently, topical antifungal therapy is primarily used adjunctively in invasive fungal sinusitis, although efficacy is difficult to determine in the literature. Topical antifungal therapy may improve objective findings such as mucosal thickening on computed tomography and endoscopic examination, but does not improve symptoms over placebo in CRS patients.[57] Future studies should examine use of topical antifungals in patients with allergic fungal sinusitis. Topical antifungals may be an option for refractory disease in this population and seem to have a low risk profile.[61]

SUMMARY

Topical therapies continually evolve as we develop our understanding of the multifactorial etiologies of inflammation seen in CRS. Currently, the primary topical therapy for CRS includes saline and corticosteroids. Topical saline adjunctively improves symptoms and likely improves absorption of corticosteroids by improving mucociliary clearance. Topical corticosteroids improve symptoms in patients with and without polyps. Optimal drug, dosage, and delivery should be directed by the patient's tolerance of adverse effects and the presence of steroid-dependent medical comorbidities such as asthma. Topical antibiotics should be used in a culture-directed manner and may be helpful in treating methicillin-resistant *S aureus*–positive exacerbations. Topical antifungal therapy has generally fallen out of favor, but may be a helpful adjunctive treatment in invasive fungal sinusitis.

REFERENCES

1. Ho EY, Cady KA, Robles JS. A case study of the neti pot's rise, Americanization, and rupture as integrative medicine in U.S. media discourse. Health Commun 2016;31(10):1181–92.
2. Pynnonen MA, Mukerji SS, Kim HM, et al. Nasal saline for chronic sinonasal symptoms: a randomized controlled trial. Arch Otolaryngol Head Neck Surg 2007;133(11):1115–20.
3. Hauptman G, Ryan MW. The effect of saline solutions on nasal patency and mucociliary clearance in rhinosinusitis patients. Otolaryngol Head Neck Surg 2007; 137(5):815–21.
4. Thomas WW 3rd, Harvey RJ, Rudmik L, et al. Distribution of topical agents to the paranasal sinuses: an evidence-based review with recommendations. Int Forum Allergy Rhinol 2013;3(9):691–703.
5. Harvey R, Hannan SA, Badia L, et al. Nasal saline irrigations for the symptoms of chronic rhinosinusitis. Cochrane Database Syst Rev 2007;(3):CD006394.
6. Wei CC, Adappa ND, Cohen NA. Use of topical nasal therapies in the management of chronic rhinosinusitis. Laryngoscope 2013;123(10):2347–59.
7. Rudmik L, Soler ZM. Medical therapies for adult chronic sinusitis: a systematic review. JAMA 2015;314(9):926–39.
8. Rudmik L, Soler ZM, Orlandi RR, et al. Early postoperative care following endoscopic sinus surgery: an evidence-based review with recommendations. Int Forum Allergy Rhinol 2011;1(6):417–30.
9. Liang KL, Su MC, Tseng HC, et al. Impact of pulsatile nasal irrigation on the prognosis of functional endoscopic sinus surgery. J Otolaryngol Head Neck Surg 2008;37(2):148–53.
10. Lewenza S, Charron-Mazenod L, Cho JJ, et al. Identification of bacterial contaminants in sinus irrigation bottles from chronic rhinosinusitis patients. J Otolaryngol Head Neck Surg 2010;39(4):458–63.
11. Lee JM, Nayak JV, Doghramji LL, et al. Assessing the risk of irrigation bottle and fluid contamination after endoscopic sinus surgery. Am J Rhinol Allergy 2010; 24(3):197–9.

12. Liu CM, Kohanski MA, Mendiola M, et al. Impact of saline irrigation and topical corticosteroids on the postsurgical sinonasal microbiota. Int Forum Allergy Rhinol 2015;5(3):185–90.
13. Siddiqui R, Khan NA. Primary amoebic meningoencephalitis caused by Naegleria fowleri: an old enemy presenting new challenges. PLoS Negl Trop Dis 2014; 8(8):e3017.
14. Sittig M. William Andrew publishing. Pharmaceutical manufacturing encyclopedia. 3rd edition. Norwich (NY): William Andrew Pub; 2007.
15. Nieman L. Epidemiology and clinical manifestations of Cushing's syndrome. In: Lacroix A, editor. UpToDate. Waltham (MA): Available at: http://www.uptodate.com/contents/epidemiology-and-clinical-manifestations-of-cushings-syndrome?source=search_result&search=cushing%27s+syndrome&selectedTitle=2%7E150; Accessed June 6, 2016.
16. DelGaudio JM, Wise SK. Topical steroid drops for the treatment of sinus ostia stenosis in the postoperative period. Am J Rhinol 2006;20(6):563–7.
17. Thamboo A, Manji J, Szeitz A, et al. The safety and efficacy of short-term budesonide delivered via mucosal atomization device for chronic rhinosinusitis without nasal polyposis. Int Forum Allergy Rhinol 2014;4(5):397–402.
18. Barnes PJ. Mechanisms and resistance in glucocorticoid control of inflammation. J Steroid Biochem Mol Biol 2010;120(2–3):76–85.
19. Barnes PJ. Corticosteroid effects on cell signalling. Eur Respir J 2006;27(2): 413–26.
20. Joe SA, Thambi R, Huang J. A systematic review of the use of intranasal steroids in the treatment of chronic rhinosinusitis. Otolaryngol Head Neck Surg 2008; 139(3):340–7.
21. Banglawala SM, Oyer SL, Lohia S, et al. Olfactory outcomes in chronic rhinosinusitis with nasal polyposis after medical treatments: a systematic review and meta-analysis. Int Forum Allergy Rhinol 2014;4(12):986–94.
22. Kalish LH, Arendts G, Sacks R, et al. Topical steroids in chronic rhinosinusitis without polyps: a systematic review and meta-analysis. Otolaryngol Head Neck Surg 2009;141(6):674–83.
23. Snidvongs K, Kalish L, Sacks R, et al. Topical steroid for chronic rhinosinusitis without polyps. Cochrane Database Syst Rev 2011;(8):CD009274.
24. Chong LY, Head K, Hopkins C, et al. Intranasal steroids versus placebo or no intervention for chronic rhinosinusitis. Cochrane Database Syst Rev 2016;(4):CD011996.
25. Chong LY, Head K, Hopkins C, et al. Different types of intranasal steroids for chronic rhinosinusitis. Cochrane Database Syst Rev 2016;(4):CD011993.
26. Orlandi RR, Hwang PH. Perioperative care for advanced rhinology procedures. Otolaryngol Clin North Am 2006;39(3):463–73, viii.
27. Ratner PH, Miller SD, Hampel FC Jr, et al. Once-daily treatment with beclomethasone dipropionate nasal aerosol does not affect hypothalamic-pituitary-adrenal axis function. Ann Allergy Asthma Immunol 2012;109(5):336–41.
28. Liang J, Strong EB. Examining the safety of prednisolone acetate 1% nasal spray for treatment of nasal polyposis. Int Forum Allergy Rhinol 2012;2(2):126–9.
29. Passali D, Spinosi MC, Crisanti A, et al. Mometasone furoate nasal spray: a systematic review. Multidiscip Respir Med 2016;11:18.
30. Lund VJ, Flood J, Sykes AP, et al. Effect of fluticasone in severe polyposis. Arch Otolaryngol Head Neck Surg 1998;124(5):513–8.
31. Neubauer PD, Schwam ZG, Manes RP. Comparison of intranasal fluticasone spray, budesonide atomizer, and budesonide respules in patients with chronic

rhinosinusitis with polyposis after endoscopic sinus surgery. Int Forum Allergy Rhinol 2016;6(3):233–7.

32. Mygind N. Upper airway: structure, function and therapy. In: Moren F, Newhouse MT, Dolovich MB, editors. Aerosols in medicine. Principles, diagnosis, and therapy. Amsterdam (Netherlands): Elsevier; 1985. p. 1–20.

33. Moffett AJ. Nasal analgesia by postural instillation. Anaesthesia 1947;2(1):31–4.

34. Habib AR, Thamboo A, Manji J, et al. The effect of head position on the distribution of topical nasal medication using the Mucosal Atomization Device: a cadaver study. Int Forum Allergy Rhinol 2013;3(12):958–62.

35. Tran KN, Beule AG, Singal D, et al. Frontal ostium restenosis after the endoscopic modified Lothrop procedure. Laryngoscope 2007;117(8):1457–62.

36. Smith TL. The endoscopic modified Lothrop procedure: finally ready for prime time in the management of inflammatory sinus disease. Int Forum Allergy Rhinol 2016;6(5):549.

37. Schulze SL, Loehrl TA, Smith TL. Outcomes of the modified endoscopic Lothrop procedure. Am J Rhinol 2002;16(5):269–73.

38. Cannady SB, Batra PS, Citardi MJ, et al. Comparison of delivery of topical medications to the paranasal sinuses via "vertex-to-floor" position and atomizer spray after FESS. Otolaryngol Head Neck Surg 2005;133(5):735–40.

39. Naidoo Y, Bassiouni A, Keen M, et al. Long-term outcomes for the endoscopic modified Lothrop/Draf III procedure: a 10-year review. Laryngoscope 2014; 124(1):43–9.

40. Salib RJ, Howarth PH. Safety and tolerability profiles of intranasal antihistamines and intranasal corticosteroids in the treatment of allergic rhinitis. Drug Saf 2003; 26(12):863–93.

41. Mullol J, Obando A, Pujols L, et al. Corticosteroid treatment in chronic rhinosinusitis: the possibilities and the limits. Immunol Allergy Clin North Am 2009;29(4): 657–68.

42. Seiberling KA, Chang DF, Nyirady J, et al. Effect of intranasal budesonide irrigations on intraocular pressure. Int Forum Allergy Rhinol 2013;3(9):704–7.

43. Soudry E, Wang J, Vaezeafshar R, et al. Safety analysis of long-term budesonide nasal irrigations in patients with chronic rhinosinusitis post endoscopic sinus surgery. Int Forum Allergy Rhinol 2016;6(6):568–72.

44. Silverman M, Sheffer A, Diaz PV, et al. Outcome of pregnancy in a randomized controlled study of patients with asthma exposed to budesonide. Ann Allergy Asthma Immunol 2005;95(6):566–70.

45. Ellegard EK, Hellgren M, Karlsson NG. Fluticasone propionate aqueous nasal spray in pregnancy rhinitis. Clin Otolaryngol Allied Sci 2001;26(5):394–400.

46. Kennedy JL, Borish L. Chronic rhinosinusitis and antibiotics: the good, the bad, and the ugly. Am J Rhinol Allergy 2013;27(6):467–72.

47. Vaughan WC, Carvalho G. Use of nebulized antibiotics for acute infections in chronic sinusitis. Otolaryngol Head Neck Surg 2002;127(6):558–68.

48. Soler ZM, Oyer SL, Kern RC, et al. Antimicrobials and chronic rhinosinusitis with or without polyposis in adults: an evidenced-based review with recommendations. Int Forum Allergy Rhinol 2013;3(1):31–47.

49. Ammerlaan HS, Kluytmans JA, Wertheim HF, et al. Eradication of methicillin-resistant Staphylococcus aureus carriage: a systematic review. Clin Infect Dis 2009;48(7):922–30.

50. Ha KR, Psaltis AJ, Butcher AR, et al. In vitro activity of mupirocin on clinical isolates of Staphylococcus aureus and its potential implications in chronic rhinosinusitis. Laryngoscope 2008;118(3):535–40.

51. Rosenfeld M, Gibson R, McNamara S, et al. Serum and lower respiratory tract drug concentrations after tobramycin inhalation in young children with cystic fibrosis. J Pediatr 2001;139(4):572–7.

52. Moss RB, King VV. Management of sinusitis in cystic fibrosis by endoscopic surgery and serial antimicrobial lavage. Reduction in recurrence requiring surgery. Arch Otolaryngol Head Neck Surg 1995;121(5):566–72.

53. Ponikau JU, Sherris DA, Kern EB, et al. The diagnosis and incidence of allergic fungal sinusitis. Mayo Clin Proc 1999;74(9):877–84.

54. Weschta M, Rimek D, Formanek M, et al. Topical antifungal treatment of chronic rhinosinusitis with nasal polyps: a randomized, double-blind clinical trial. J Allergy Clin Immunol 2004;113(6):1122–8.

55. Ricchetti A, Landis BN, Maffioli A, et al. Effect of anti-fungal nasal lavage with amphotericin B on nasal polyposis. J Laryngol Otol 2002;116(4):261–3.

56. Ponikau JU, Sherris DA, Kita H, et al. Intranasal antifungal treatment in 51 patients with chronic rhinosinusitis. J Allergy Clin Immunol 2002;110(6):862–6.

57. Ponikau JU, Sherris DA, Weaver A, et al. Treatment of chronic rhinosinusitis with intranasal amphotericin B: a randomized, placebo-controlled, double-blind pilot trial. J Allergy Clin Immunol 2005;115(1):125–31.

58. Ebbens FA, Scadding GK, Badia L, et al. Amphotericin B nasal lavages: not a solution for patients with chronic rhinosinusitis. J Allergy Clin Immunol 2006;118(5): 1149–56.

59. Isaacs S, Fakhri S, Luong A, et al. A meta-analysis of topical amphotericin B for the treatment of chronic rhinosinusitis. Int Forum Allergy Rhinol 2011;1(4):250–4.

60. Sacks PL 4th, Harvey RJ, Rimmer J, et al. Antifungal therapy in the treatment of chronic rhinosinusitis: a meta-analysis. Am J Rhinol Allergy 2012;26(2):141–7.

61. Gan EC, Thamboo A, Rudmik L, et al. Medical management of allergic fungal rhinosinusitis following endoscopic sinus surgery: an evidence-based review and recommendations. Int Forum Allergy Rhinol 2014;4(9):702–15.

Advances in Absorbable Biomaterials and Nasal Packing

Conner J. Massey, MD[a], Ameet Singh, MD[b],*

KEYWORDS

- Nasal biomaterials • Absorbable • Removable • Packing • Sinus surgery
- Chronic rhinosinusitis

KEY POINTS

- A nasal biomaterial should function to promote wound healing, prevent hemorrhage, and minimize patient discomfort.
- A vast number of nasal biomaterials exist, and have been studied to varying degrees.
- Nonabsorbable nasal packing is associated with greater patient discomfort compared with absorbable packs given that the pack must be removed during the postoperative period.
- Interstudy comparison of nasal biomaterials is difficult because of the wide variety of evaluation methods.
- Consensus must be established regarding the optimal method of assessing nasal biomaterial performance before further trials are undertaken.

INTRODUCTION

Biomaterials have played an increasingly vital role in otolaryngology since the first description of the tympanostomy tube in the 1850s. Reliance on these powerful clinical tools has mirrored the increase in their sophistication, ease of use, and mass manufacture. This phenomenon is aptly reflected by the development and implementation of nasal biomaterials and packing for use in functional endoscopic sinus surgery (FESS), an area that has seen many different products become available over the past 50 years.

Disclosures: A. Singh has received research grants from Intersect ENT and Johnson & Johnson, and has worked as a consultant for Lannett Pharmaceuticals and Intersect ENT.
[a] Department of Otolaryngology, University of Colorado School of Medicine, 12631 East 17th Avenue, B-205, Aurora, CO 80045, USA; [b] Rhinology & Skull Base Surgery, Division of Otolaryngology–Head and Neck Surgery, The George Washington University School of Medicine, 2300 M Street Northwest, 4th Floor, Washington, DC 20037, USA
* Corresponding author.
E-mail address: dr.ameetsingh.ent@gmail.com

Otolaryngol Clin N Am 50 (2017) 545–563
http://dx.doi.org/10.1016/j.otc.2017.01.006
0030-6665/17/© 2017 Elsevier Inc. All rights reserved.

oto.theclinics.com

FESS has several common but troublesome adverse outcomes that nasal biomaterials have been developed to either overcome or prevent. In particular, nasal packing serves to achieve the following goals:

1. Promote hemostasis
2. Allow or enhance proper wound healing
3. Maintain patient comfort
4. Reduce inflammation through drug delivery

Intraoperative and postoperative hemorrhage are common complications in FESS.[1] Nasal biomaterials have been designed to address this problem through enzymatic activation of the coagulation cascade, physical pressure tamponade, or both. In clinical trials, hemostatic performance has been assessed via several different metrics, including patient-reported blood loss, weight of blood loss, volume of blood loss, bleeding time, incidence of postoperative hemorrhage, need for repacking, and custom and validated bleeding scales.

Adhesions are another frequently encountered complication after FESS. Estimated to occur in roughly a third of patients,[2] these undesirable surgical outcomes may impair mucociliary clearance, prevent topical drug delivery, increase the need for postoperative interventions, and lead to recurrence of chronic rhinosinusitis symptoms, particularly when adhesions occur between the middle turbinate and the lateral nasal wall. Rhinologic compounds prevent adhesions and scarring by acting as spacers that ensure middle turbinate medialization during the healing process. They may also be used as stents that maintain sinus ostial patency. Certain biomaterials are posited to enhance wound healing on a biochemical level as well. There is currently no clinical standard for assessing the wound healing properties of a given biomaterial. Various outcomes assessed in clinical trials include endoscopic evaluation of adhesions, granulation tissue, crusting, and ostial patency, as well as mucosal biopsy. Investigators have used validated endoscopic scoring systems, such as the Lund-Kennedy system, or have created their own custom endoscopic scores.

Although biomaterials are often used after FESS to prevent hemorrhage and adhesion formation, it is often at the expense of patient comfort. Nasal packing exacerbates postoperative nasal obstruction and facial pressure, and its removal is sometimes considered to be more traumatic than the surgery.[3] Absorbable biomaterials have been developed to avoid the need to pull nasal packs and thereby decrease patient discomfort. However, any type of nasal packing inserted after FESS likely contributes to patient discomfort to some degree. In clinical trials, patient discomfort associated with nasal packing use is most commonly assessed with a visual analog scale (VAS), either while the pack is in situ or at the time of its removal.

In addition, a substantial amount of energy has been devoted to developing nasal biomaterials capable of topical corticosteroid delivery to the paranasal tissues. Such a product ideally prevents disease recurrence and lessens the need for systemic medical therapy. This important topic is covered in depth elsewhere in this issue.

This article evaluates how various nasal biomaterials perform with respect to hemostasis, wound healing, and patient comfort. The conclusions were derived only from prospective, randomized controlled trials (RCTs) conducted in humans. Biomaterials are presented and discussed in order, as shown in **Fig. 1**.

NONABSORBABLE PACKING

Used in sinus surgery for decades, nonabsorbable packing generally takes the form of a foam tampon or sponge that is inserted into the middle meatus or nasal cavity

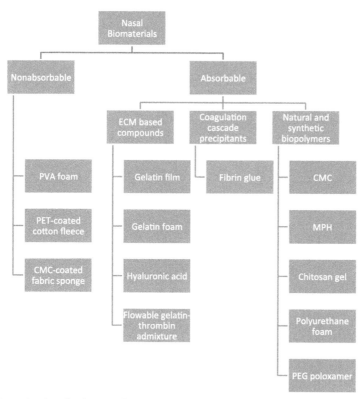

Fig. 1. Organizational schema of nasal biomaterials. CMC, carboxymethylcellulose; ECM, extracellular matrix; MPH, microporous polysaccharide hemospheres; PEG, polyethylene glycol; PET, polyethylene terephthalate; PVA, polyvinyl acetate.

immediately following surgery. It is designed to serve as a physical barrier between the middle meatus and lateral nasal wall, as well as being a hemostatic agent that acts mainly via pressure tamponade. Various coatings and sheaths have been developed that either increase the hemostatic potential or allow more facile extraction during postoperative visits. This article focuses on some of the most widely available products currently in use, including polyvinyl acetate (PVA) foam (Merocel, Medtronic Xomed, Jacksonville, FL), polyethylene terephthalate–coated cotton fleece (Telfa, The Kendall Company, Boston, MA), and carboxymethylcellulose (CMC)-coated fabric tampons (Rapid Rhino Riemann, Applied Therapeutics, Obernberg, Germany) (**Table 1**).

As shown by many of the studies collected here, PVA is often the standard with which other biomaterials are compared. The product is available as a standard foam tampon for insertion into the middle meatus, as well as with manufacturer-applied coatings such as polyethylene film (Merocel 2000, Medtronic Xomed) and oxidized cellulose (Merocel Hemox, Medtronic Xomed). In a single-blind trial, Melis and colleagues[4] compared the 2 coated PVA sponges with uncoated PVA. The packs were evaluated for hemostasis and pain on pack removal. The standard PVA pack performed significantly worse for hemostasis on pack removal, whereas the oxidized cellulose pack performed best. The polyethylene film pack was associated with the least patient discomfort on extraction.

Table 1
Nonabsorbable nasal packs

	Study	Study Size (n)	Comparison Method	Comparison	Patient Comfort (Outcome Measure)	Hemostasis (Outcome Measure)	Wound Healing (Outcome Measure)
PVA foam	Melis et al,[4] 2015	90	Interpatient	pePVA	Favors pePVA (VAS on pack removal)	Favors pePVA (bleeding score on pack removal)	NA
				ocPVA	Favors ocPVA (VAS on pack removal)	Favors ocPVA (bleeding score on pack removal)	NA
	Cho et al,[15] 2013	100	Intrapatient	Gelatin foam	Favors gelatin foam (VAS while in situ)	Favors gelatin foam (bleeding score on pack removal)	Equivalent (Lund-Kennedy)
	Miller et al,[20] 2003	37	Intrapatient	HA	NA	NA	Equivalent (adhesions)
	Franklin & Wright,[21] 2007	35	Intrapatient	HA	NA	NA	Equivalent (endoscopic score)
	Berlucchi et al,[22] 2009	66[a]	Not stated	HA	NA	NA	Favors HA (adhesions)
	Vaiman et al,[28] 2005	64	Interpatient	Fibrin glue	NA	Favors fibrin glue (postoperative bleeding episodes)	NA
	Yu et al,[29] 2014	41	Intrapatient	Fibrin glue	Favors fibrin glue (VAS on pack removal)	NA	Favors fibrin glue (eg, adhesions, crusting)
	Al-Shaikh et al,[31] 2014	50	Intrapatient	OCP	Favors OCP (VAS)	Favors OCP (bleeding score)	Equivalent (adhesions)
	Verim et al,[42] 2014	56	Intrapatient	PUF	Favors PUF (VAS)	NA	Equivalent (Lund-Kennedy)

	Study	No.	Comparison	Material	Pain	Bleeding	Endoscopy/Other
Glove finger sheathed PVA	Kim et al,[5] 2012	30	Interpatient	PVA	Favors glove-sheathed PVA (VAS)	Favors glove-sheathed PVA (weight of blood loss)	Favors glove-sheathed PVA (Lund-Kennedy)
	Akbari et al,[6] 2012	37	Intrapatient	PVA	Favors glove-sheathed PVA (VAS on pack removal)	NA	Equivalent (mucosal inflammation on biopsy)
	Shoman et al,[41] 2009	30	Intrapatient	PUF	Equivalent (VAS)	Equivalent (bleeding score)	Equivalent (adhesions, mucosal edema)
	Szczygielski et al,[34] 2010	60	Interpatient	CMC	Favors CMC (VAS)	Equivalent (postoperative bleeding requiring repacking)	Equivalent (adhesions)
PET-coated cotton fleece	Cruise et al,[7] 2009	45	Intrapatient	CMC-coated fabric sponge	Favors CMC-coated fabric sponge (VAS on removal)	Equivalent (amount of bleeding on removal)	Equivalent (Lund-Kennedy)

Abbreviations: HA, hyaluronic acid; NA, not available; OCP, oxidized cellulose powder; ocPVA, oxidized cellulose-coated PVA; pePVA, polyethylene film PVA; PET, polyethylene terephthalate; PUF, polyurethane foam; VAS, visual analog scale.
[a] Treatments were randomized to 88 nasal cavities in 66 patients.

Several studies have examined PVA sheathed in a vinyl or latex glove finger. Kim and colleagues[5] showed that PVA sheathed in a latex glove finger was significantly more comfortable, and reduced bleeding on pack removal compared with standard PVA. The investigators also examined wound healing via Lund-Kennedy endoscopic scoring, and found that the glove-sheathed PVA performed significantly better. Akbari and colleagues[6] also studied glove finger–sheathed PVA, finding similar results for comfort compared with plain PVA. Wound healing, as shown via inflammation seen on mucosal biopsy, was equivalent for both packs. The investigators did not specify the type of glove material that was used.

Polyethylene terephthalate–coated cotton fleece has been compared with a CMC-coated fabric sponge in a double-blind study. Both products performed similarly for wound healing and hemostasis, although the CMC-coated fabric sponge caused significantly less pain on removal.[7]

Although nonabsorbable nasal packs like PVA have long been considered standard of care after FESS, several significant drawbacks have caused them to lose popularity among sinus surgeons. Most of the issues arise from packing removal during the early postoperative period, which is a traumatic event because the packs swell significantly as they absorb blood and secretions. Not only does pack extraction cause significant discomfort to the patient, it may potentiate hemorrhage and induce mucosal shearing. The pressure exerted by the pack expansion may contribute to significant demucosalization, which has been estimated to be as much as 70% in the region of the pack.[8] Other complications and side effects of nonabsorbable packing include obstructive sleep apnea, eustachian tube dysfunction,[9] posterior dislodgement and aspiration,[10] and toxic shock syndrome.[11] Taken together, these adverse features have driven the development of bioabsorbable nasal materials that perform many of the same functions as nonabsorbable packing, but dissolve and fragment over time.

ABSORBABLE BIOMATERIALS

Absorbable nasal biomaterials encompass a multitude of compounds that exert their functions over a limited period of time until their natural dissolution in the nasal cavity occurs. Taking a wide variety of forms, including foams, gels, meshes, flowable matrices, films, and powders, these materials are composed of an equally diverse array of substances. This article categorizes and discusses the absorbable biomaterials based on their chemical composition, organized as follows:

- Extracellular matrix (ECM)–based compounds
- Coagulation cascade precipitants
- Natural and synthetic biopolymers

Extracellular Matrix–based Compounds

ECM-based compounds are either derived from collagen or hyaluronic acid (HA). These substances are generally bovine or porcine in origin, and can be formulated as films, sponges, gels, and meshes that are rapidly reabsorbed by the body (**Table 2**).

Collagen-based compounds

Collagen in surgical biomaterials usually takes the form of bovine-derived or porcine-derived gelatin. This protein is rapidly phagocytosed and enzymatically degraded, achieving total liquefaction in 3 to 5 days. As a class, collagen-based biomaterials exert their hemostatic properties through 2 mechanisms. When formulated as a porous sponge, these materials expand on contact with blood, resulting in pressure tamponade. Collagen also precipitates the coagulation cascade via the intrinsic pathway, a process that is further amplified when admixed with thrombin.

Collagen biomaterials have been variably studied in the setting of FESS. A single RCT exists examining the utility of gelatin film (Gelfilm, Pharmacia and Upjohn Company, Kalamazoo, MI).[12] Using a pediatric population, the investigators used this material as a middle meatal stent and examined wound healing outcomes. No significant differences were seen in adhesions, granulation tissue, or sinus ostial patency between middle meati stented with gelatin film and those without stenting.

Collagen is also available as a foam or sponge, of which several proprietary formulations are commercially available. Although these products may possess similar hemostatic and wound healing properties, they differ with regard to density and porosity. Gelfoam (Pharmacia and Upjohn Company) has been evaluated against an unpacked control.[13] After soaking the material in Terramycin ointment, the sponges were placed in the middle meatus. No differences were seen between the packed sides and the unpacked sides in terms of crusting, granulation tissue, edema, or patient comfort. Cutanplast (Mascia Brunelli SpA, Milan, Italy) has been compared with PVA, as well as another proprietary gelatin foam product, Spongostan (Ferrosan, Copenhagen, Denmark). The two gelatin foam products produced equivalent Lund-Kennedy scores and bleeding scores, although Cutanplast was more comfortable for patients.[14] Cutanplast performed better than PVA for hemostasis and comfort, but Lund-Kennedy scores were equal for both products.[15]

Collagen compounds can also be prepared with thrombin for increased hemostatic effect. A flowable admixture of thrombin and granulated gelatin (FloSeal, Baxter International, Deerfield, IL) has been developed as a surgical hemostatic agent. Although this gelatin-thrombin admixture has been shown to reduce intraoperative and postoperative hemorrhage compared with unpacked control,[16] controversy exists over the effects this material exerts on wound healing. An often-cited animal study by Maccabee and colleagues[17] found that the flowable gelatin-thrombin admixture became incorporated into the sinus mucosa. The investigators stripped the entire mucosa of the maxillary sinus of rabbits, which were then filled with the compound and sealed. This methodology serves as a poor model for how this material is used in sinus surgery, so the conclusions should be interpreted accordingly.

Chandra and colleagues[18] compared flowable gelatin-thrombin admixture with thrombin-soaked gelatin sponge. Although these compounds had equivalent hemostatic capabilities, the gelatin-thrombin admixture treatment arm had significantly more adhesions and granulation tissue. In a subsequent article, the investigators followed each cohort retrospectively, showing that ethmoidal cavities receiving the gelatin-thrombin admixture had more adhesions and required more lysis interventions postoperatively than the thrombin-soaked gelatin sponge treatment side.[19] Histologic analysis of adhesion in 1 patient packed with gelatin-thrombin admixture showed incorporation of foreign material. The investigators concluded that the pastelike consistency of this biomaterial lacked significant rigidity for middle meatal stenting.

Collagen biomaterials in general seem to be effective hemostatic agents, although their wound healing properties have not been shown consistently among available RCTs. Although the addition of thrombin may increase their hemostatic potential, controversy exists over whether collagen-thrombin compounds cause adverse wound healing outcomes.

Hyaluronic acid biomaterials

As a surgical dressing, HA compounds are thought to increase the rate of reepithelialization in the wound bed. For FESS applications, they have been formulated as gels,

Table 2
Extracellular matrix-based compounds

	Study	Study Size (n)	Comparison Method	Comparison	Patient Comfort (Outcome Measure)	Hemostasis (Outcome Measure)	Wound Healing (Outcome Measure)
Gelatin film	Tom et al,[12] 1997	51	Intrapatient	Unpacked control	NA	NA	Equivalent (adhesions, granulation tissue, ostial patency)
Gelatin foam	Wee et al,[13] 2012	21	Intrapatient	Unpacked control	Equivalent (symptom index)	NA	Equivalent (eg, adhesions, crusting, edema)
	Cho et al,[14] 2015 (Cutanplast)	100	Intrapatient	Gelatin foam (Spongostan)	Favors Cutanplast (symptom index)	Equivalent (bleeding scale)	Equivalent (Lund-Kennedy)
	Cho et al,[15] 2013	100	Intrapatient	PVA	Favors gelatin foam (VAS)	Favors gelatin foam (bleeding scale on pack removal)	Equivalent (Lund-Kennedy)
Flowable gelatin-thrombin admixture	Jameson et al,[16] 2006	45	Intrapatient	Unpacked control	Favors gelatin-thrombin admixture (pain relative to contralateral side)	Favors gelatin-thrombin admixture (postoperative bleeding time)	Equivalent (crusting and scarring)
	Beyea & Rotenberg,[38] 2011	18	Interpatient	MPH	NA	Equivalent (intraoperative blood loss amount)	NA
	Chandra et al,[18] 2003	20	Intrapatient	Thrombin-soaked gelatin foam	NA	Equivalent (need for additional packing)	Favors thrombin-soaked gelatin foam (adhesions, granulation tissue)

	Study	N	Comparison	Comparator			
HA	Miller et al,[20] 2003	37	Intrapatient	PVA	NA	NA	Equivalent (adhesions, edema)
	Franklin & Castel,[21] 2007	35	Intrapatient	PVA	NA	NA	Equivalent (endoscopic score)
	Berlucchi et al,[22] 2009	66[a]	Not stated	PVA	NA	NA	Favors HA (adhesions)
	Wormald et al,[23] 2006	42	Intrapatient	Unpacked control	NA	NA	Equivalent (adhesions, edema)
	Kimmelman et al,[25] 2001	10	Intrapatient	Unpacked control	Favors HA (VAS)	NA	Favors HA (adhesions, middle meatal stenosis)
	Frenkiel et al,[26] 2002	20	Intrapatient	Unpacked control	NA	Equivalent (bleeding scale, volume of blood loss)	NA
	Shi et al,[27] 2013	54	Intrapatient	Unpacked control	NA	NA	Favors HA (eg, adhesions, crusts)
	Song et al,[44] 2013	66	Intrapatient	PEG poloxamer	NA	NA	Equivalent (adhesions, edema)
HA-collagen hybrid	Hu et al,[24] 2008	60	Intrapatient	Unpacked control	NA	Favors HA-collagen hybrid (incidence of postoperative bleeds)	Equivalent (eg, adhesions, granulation tissue)

Abbreviations: MPH, microporous polysaccharide hemospheres; PEG, polyethylene glycol.
[a] Treatments were randomized to 88 nasal cavities in 66 patients.

foams, and meshes. HA has also been combined with collagen to create a hybrid foam sponge.

Among the available HA products, an esterified HA nasal pack (MeroGel, Medtronic Xomed) has undergone the most extensive evaluation. Three studies have compared esterified HA packs with PVA. Miller and colleagues[20] and Franklin and Wright[21] found similar rates for adhesions and endoscopic scores between esterified HA packs and PVA. For Berlucchi and colleagues,[22] esterified HA performed better than PVA with respect to preventing adhesions at 4 and 12 weeks postoperatively. Esterified HA packs have also been compared with unpacked control, and no significant differences were seen between treatment arms in terms of adhesions or edema.[23]

The efficacy of an HA-collagen hybrid pack composed of 80% collagen and 20% HA (MeroPack, Medtronic Xomed) was evaluated in 60 pediatric patients.[24] Compared with unpacked control, the investigators found that this hybrid pack significantly reduced the incidence of postoperative hemorrhage. No differences were seen between treatment arms with respect to adhesions, granulation tissue, and sinus ostial patency at 8 and 12 weeks postoperatively.

Two studies have compared a cross-linked, water-insoluble HA polymer gel (Sepragel Sinus, Genzyme Biosurgery, Cambridge, MA) with unpacked control. In a study of 10 patients with intrapatient control, HA gel was randomized to a single ethmoidectomy cavity and then evaluated at 1-week intervals, and more HA gel was added to the cavity during postoperative visits at the surgeon's discretion.[25] The use of HA gel was associated with significantly reduced adhesions, granulation tissue, edema, and middle meatal stenosis, as well as improved postoperative comfort. However, patients and evaluators were not blinded to treatment arms. The hemostatic properties of this compound were studied by Frenkiel and colleagues,[26] and treatment arms were found to be equivalent for volume of blood loss, but nonblinded evaluators thought that HA gel provided either effective or very effective hemostasis in 95% of cavities.

A newer agent in this class, cross-linked hyaluronan hydrogel (PureRegen Gel Sinus, BioRegen Biomedical, Changzhou, China), has been evaluated against unpacked control in a single trial.[27] This material showed improved reepithelialization at 2, 4, and 8 weeks postoperatively as determined via endoscopic score.

HA products seem to confer modest benefit with respect to wound healing. Esterified HA packs have performed inconsistently over multiple trials. Cross-linked HA gel and hyaluronan hydrogel seem to have performed better, although only single studies exist for each. The hemostatic properties of HA biomaterials have not been established.

COAGULATION CASCADE PRECIPITANTS

These agents are composed primarily of pooled human-origin blood products that activate the coagulation cascade, of which fibrin glue (Tisseel, Baxter Healthcare Corp, Deerfield, IL) is the sole member of its class (**Table 3**). Formulated as a gel, this material is derived from purified fibrinogen and thrombin that, when mixed, leads to clot formation when applied at the site of hemorrhage.

Two trials have studied the efficacy of fibrin glue in FESS, both comparing this material with PVA. Vaiman and colleagues[28] found that fibrin glue was more effective than PVA for hemostasis by measuring outcomes such as bleeding after pack removal and late postoperative hemorrhage. Fibrin glue performed better in that it did not cause bleeding on pack removal, although there was 1 episode of late postoperative hemorrhage in the fibrin glue group, which was not seen with PVA. Yu and colleagues[29] assessed the wound healing properties of fibrin glue. Refuting earlier animal studies

Table 3
Coagulation cascade precipitants

Study	Study Size (n)	Comparison Method	Comparison	Patient Comfort (Outcome Measure)	Hemostasis (Outcome Measure)	Wound Healing (Outcome Measure)
Fibrin glue						
Vaiman et al,[28] 2005	64	Interpatient	PVA	NA	Favors fibrin glue (postoperative bleeding episodes)	NA
Yu et al,[29] 2014	41	Intrapatient	PVA	Favors fibrin glue (VAS on pack removal)	NA	Favors fibrin glue (eg, adhesions, crusting)

that suggested proinflammatory properties of fibrin glue on sinonasal mucosa,[30] the investigators showed that this material was associated with a lesser degree of crusting, granulation tissue, and adhesions compared with PVA. Patients also noted less pain on pack removal with fibrin glue.

These 2 trials suggest that fibrin glue shows superior wound healing and hemostatic properties compared with PVA, although the product has not been trialed against unpacked control or other absorbable biomaterials.

NATURAL AND SYNTHETIC BIOPOLYMERS

Biomaterials in this class are composed of a diverse set of compounds that are either natural or synthetic in origin (**Table 4**). Naturally derived materials include oxidized cellulose, CMC, and microporous polysaccharide hemospheres (MPH), as well as the crustacean-derived biopolymer, chitosan. Synthetic materials formulated for use in FESS include polyurethane and polyethylene glycol (PEG).

Despite being one of the earliest bioabsorbable compounds to be used for hemostasis in rhinology, oxidized cellulose has only been trialed in a single RCT to date. This material promotes hemostasis via platelet aggregation. In a study of 50 patients, Al-Shaikh and colleagues[31] compared a powdered formulation of oxidized cellulose (Bloodcare, Anser Medical, Saffron Walden, United Kingdom) with PVA. Although the degree of adhesions was equivalent for both products, the oxidized cellulose powder performed better with respect to hemostasis and comfort in the first 24 hours after surgery.

Another plant-derived product, CMC (Sinufoam, Arthrocare, Austin, TX), acts in a similar fashion to oxidized cellulose, and may be formulated as a gel, mesh, or foam. Four RCTs conducted on this material have shown inconsistent performance with respect to hemostasis and wound healing. Compared with unpacked control, CMC did not significantly reduce intraoperative or postoperative bleeding scores.[32] In a separate study, the same group of investigators showed that CMC produced similar degrees of crusting, adhesions, and reepithelialization compared with unpacked control.[33] CMC was also compared with latex glove–sheathed PVA, and hemostasis and wound healing properties were similar for both packs, although CMC was more comfortable.[34] In addition, CMC has also been evaluated against 2 other plant-based polysaccharide products: MPH (Arista, Medafor Inc, Minneapolis, MN) and a potato starch foam wafer (Nexfoam, Hemostasis LLC, St Paul, MN).[35] In this trial, no significant differences were seen between all products in terms of patient-reported bleeding or pain during the postoperative period. Wound healing parameters such as adhesions, edema, and granulation tissue, were equivalent for all products.

MPH is a potato starch–sourced hemostatic agent that is formulated as an injectable powder. Two studies have compared MPH with unpacked control, determining that MPH significantly improved bleeding scores on the first postoperative day,[36] but no differences were seen in terms of adhesions or edema.[37] MPH was also compared with a flowable gelatin-thrombin admixture for intraoperative blood loss, and the products were found to be similar.[38]

Chitosan, a biopolymer synthesized from crustacean-sourced chitin, is available as an aerosol or gel. The gel formulation has performed well compared with unpacked control. Valentine and colleagues[40] showed that chitosan gel reduced intraoperative bleeding as determined via Boezaart bleeding scale, but was equivalent to unpacked control for patient comfort.[39] The study further showed that chitosan gel was associated with fewer adhesions and crusts, and less granulation tissue. In a separate trial, sinus ostial patency was improved with use of the gel compared with unpacked control.

Among the first purely synthetic nasal packs to be developed for FESS, lyophilized polyurethane foam (PUF; Nasopore, Stryker, Hamilton, Canada) is designed as an absorbable middle meatal spacer. Its hydrophilic properties allow controlled fragmentation after insertion. Two trials have compared PUF with some form of nonabsorbable packing. Shoman and colleagues[41] found that PUF produced similar outcomes to PVA sheathed in a vinyl glove finger for hemostasis and patient comfort on pack removal, as well as for mucosal edema and adhesions. Compared with plain PVA, PUF was associated with a higher degree of patient comfort, but wound healing properties were similar.[42] PUF has also been trialed against unpacked controls.[43] No differences were seen between treatment arms for patient-reported blood loss during postoperative days 1 to 3; however, a significant reduction in facial pressure was seen with PUF-treated sides.

A single trial has evaluated the efficacy of a thermosensitive PEG poloxamer (TPX, Samyang Co, Seoul, South Korea) as an antiadhesion barrier that is also readily bioabsorbed.[44] All patients received PVA immediately following FESS. The PVA packs were removed at 24 hours, after which nasal cavities were randomized to receive either TPX or HA packing. The investigators observed no significant differences between the two packs with respect to reepithelialization, adhesions, or crusting. Outcomes regarding patient comfort and hemostasis were not assessed.

Plant-based biomaterials like CMC, MPH, and oxidized cellulose have been variably studied for their hemostatic and wound healing properties. The available RCTs suggest that MPH and oxidized cellulose powder have performed well with respect to hemostasis, although they have not been shown to promote wound healing. Although CMC has been the most extensively trialed plant-based material, the evidence regarding its wound healing and hemostatic properties is conflicting. A single trial has supported the use of chitosan gel as an intraoperative hemostatic agent, whereas its wound healing properties have been established in 2 separate trials. For the synthetic agents, PUF has shown similar wound healing properties to PVA, although the evidence is mixed regarding its hemostatic abilities. The newer synthetic agent TPX has shown similar wound healing outcomes to HA packing.

DISCUSSION

As shown by the studies collected in this article, a vast array of rhinologic biomaterials exist and have been studied to varying degrees. Despite the wealth of data presented here, it is difficult to ascertain the overall performance of a given biomaterial for several critical reasons. For example, it is important to consider what investigators chose to evaluate a product against. Should the ideal comparison material be unpacked control, standard nasal packing (eg, PVA), or a similar product of the same class? PVA was one of the most popular packs against which a material was trialed, although the utility of this comparison can be questioned when examining a biomaterial with vastly different physical properties. It seems obvious that a viscous bioabsorbable pack like fibrin glue will outperform PVA for certain outcomes like patient comfort, and this seems to be the case for many comparisons between absorbable and nonabsorbable packs.

Further complicating this issue, a myriad of different metrics were used to evaluate the performance of a given biomaterial, making interstudy comparison challenging. Although VASs were most commonly used to evaluate discomfort, there seems to be no standard method to assess for hemostatic and wound healing properties. Antisdel and colleagues[35] broached this issue in their recent study comparing hemostatic agents, and proposed the use of patient-reported postoperative bleeding as a

Table 4
Natural and synthetic biopolymers

	Study	Study Size (n)	Comparison Method	Comparison	Patient Comfort (Outcome Measure)	Hemostasis (Outcome Measure)	Wound Healing (Outcome Measure)
OCP	Al-Shaikh et al,[31] 2014	50	Intrapatient	PVA	Favors OCP (VAS)	Favors OCP (bleeding score)	Equivalent (adhesions)
Carboxymethylcellulose	Kastl et al,[32] 2009	41	Intrapatient	Unpacked control	NA	Equivalent (intraoperative Boezaart scale, postoperative bleeding score)	NA
	Kastl et al,[33] 2009	26	Intrapatient	Unpacked control	NA	NA	Equivalent (eg, adhesions, crusting)
	Szczygielski et al,[34] 2010	60	Interpatient	PVA sheathed latex glove finger	Favors CMC (VAS)	Equivalent (postoperative bleeding requiring repacking)	Equivalent (adhesions)
	Antisdel et al,[35] 2016	48	Intrapatient	MPH	Equivalent (VAS)	Equivalent (patient-reported bleeding score)	Equivalent (eg, adhesions, granulation tissue)
				Potato starch foam wafer	Equivalent (VAS)	Equivalent (patient-reported bleeding score)	Equivalent (eg, adhesions, granulation tissue)
Microporous polysaccharide hemospheres				Potato starch foam wafer	Equivalent (VAS)	Equivalent (patient-reported bleeding score)	Equivalent (eg, adhesions, granulation tissue)
	Antisdel et al,[36] 2009	40	Intrapatient	Unpacked control	Equivalent (VAS)	Favors MPH (bleeding score)	NA
	Antisdel et al,[37] 2011	40	Intrapatient	Unpacked control	NA	NA	Equivalent (adhesions, edema)
	Beyea & Rotenberg,[38] 2011	18	Interpatient	Flowable gelatin-thrombin admixture	NA	Equivalent (intraoperative blood loss amount)	NA

	Study	n		Control			
Chitosan gel	Valentine et al,[39] 2010	40	Intrapatient	Unpacked control	Equivalent (VAS)	Favors chitosan gel (Boezaart bleeding scale)	Favors chitosan gel (eg, edema, crusting)
	Ngoc Ha et al,[40] 2013	26	Intrapatient	Unpacked control	NA	NA	Favors chitosan gel (sinus ostial patency)
Polyurethane foam	Shoman et al,[41] 2009	30	Intrapatient	PVA sheathed in vinyl glove finger	Equivalent (VAS)	Equivalent (bleeding score)	Equivalent (adhesions, mucosal edema)
	Verim et al,[42] 2014	56	Intrapatient	PVA	Favors PUF (VAS)	NA	Equivalent (Lund-Kennedy)
	Kastl et al,[43] 2014	47	Intrapatient	Unpacked control	Favors PUF (VAS)	Equivalent (patient-reported bleeding)	NA
PEG poloxamer	Song et al,[44] 2013	54	Intrapatient	HA	NA	NA	Equivalent (eg, adhesions, crusting, edema)

standard evaluation for hemostasis. Regardless of whether this metric is optimal for the given outcome, rhinology academicians need to arrive at consensus with respect to a proper method of evaluating sinonasal biomaterials.

In addition, it is interesting to note the number of biomaterials that were found to be equivalent to unpacked control. This observation may stem either from these materials being ineffective at improving postoperative outcomes, or from routine use of nasal biomaterials after FESS not being necessary for most patients. Two retrospective studies have questioned the need for habitual nasal packing, at least with respect to control of hemorrhage after FESS. Eliashar and colleagues[45] found that packing was needed in only 8% of patients, and Orlandi and Lanza[46] yielded similar results, with 13% of patients receiving either packing or hemostatic agents after surgery.

Although this review is unable to resolve issues regarding optimal methods of evaluating nasal packing or whether packing is even needed following FESS, certain trends can be identified from the data present here. Nonabsorbable packing like PVA, long the standard biomaterial in FESS given its good hemostatic abilities, has certain drawbacks mostly inherent to the fact that the pack must be extracted at some point following surgery. This action is painful for the patient, and risks injuring mucosa and potentiating rebleeding. These problems are largely avoided with the use of bioabsorbable packing, which has performed better than nonabsorbable materials with respect to patient comfort in most of the trials presented here.

For hemostasis and wound healing outcomes, there has been a great deal of variation in performance among the absorbable biomaterials. Certain collagen-containing materials like gelatin foam and flowable gelatin pastes seem to be effective hemostatic agents, especially when compounded with thrombin. However, concerns exist as to the proinflammatory risks of using a potent activator of the coagulation cascade. Although HA compounds have been proposed to promote reepithelialization in the wound bed, the evidence supporting the wound healing abilities of these compounds is mixed. Fibrin glue has performed well compared with PVA, although further trials are needed to examine this product against unpacked control. Among the plant-derived and synthetic biomaterials with more extensive trialing, CMC and PUF have performed inconsistently, whereas MPH seems to be an effective hemostatic agent. Chitosan shows both wound healing and hemostatic properties when evaluated against unpacked control.

SUMMARY

An ideal rhinologic biomaterial should perform several vital functions when used for FESS, including hemostasis, promotion of wound healing, and maximizing patient comfort. Many biomaterials are now in use and have been evaluated to varying degrees. The observed heterogeneity in outcome measures makes the identification of superior rhinologic compounds difficult, although certain products seem to perform better than others in preventing undesirable postoperative outcomes. Consensus needs to be reached with regard to the optimal method of assessing these products before further trials are conducted.

REFERENCES

1. Hosemann W, Draf C. Danger points, complications and medico-legal aspects in endoscopic sinus surgery. GMS Curr Top Otorhinolaryngol Head Neck Surg 2013;12:Doc06.
2. Ramadan HH. Surgical causes of failure in endoscopic sinus surgery. Laryngoscope 1999;109(1):27–9.

3. Laing MR, Clark LJ. Analgesia and removal of nasal packing. Clin Otolaryngol Allied Sci 1990;15(4):339–42.

4. Melis A, Karligkiotis A, Bozzo C, et al. Comparison of three different polyvinyl alcohol packs following functional endoscopic Nasal surgery. Laryngoscope 2015;125(5):1067–71.

5. Kim DW, Lee E-J, Kim S-W, et al. Advantages of glove finger-coated polyvinyl acetate pack in endoscopic sinus surgery. Am J Rhinol Allergy 2012;26(5):e147–9.

6. Akbari E, Philpott CM, Ostry AJ, et al. A double-blind randomised controlled trial of gloved versus ungloved Merocel middle meatal spacers for endoscopic sinus surgery. Rhinology 2012;50(3):306–10.

7. Cruise AS, Amonoo-Kuofi K, Srouji I, et al. A randomized trial of Rapid Rhino Riemann and Telfa nasal packs following endoscopic sinus surgery. Clin Otolaryngol 2006;31(1):25–32.

8. Shaw CL, Dymock RB, Cowin A, et al. Effect of packing on nasal mucosa of sheep. J Laryngol Otol 2000;114(7):506–9.

9. Weber RK. Nasal packing and stenting. GMS Curr Top Otorhinolaryngol Head Neck Surg 2009;8:Doc02.

10. Hashmi SM, Gopaul SR, Prinsley PR, et al. Swallowed nasal pack: a rare but serious complication of the management of epistaxis. J Laryngol Otol 2004; 118(5):372–3.

11. Breda SD, Jacobs JB, Lebowitz AS, et al. Toxic shock syndrome in nasal surgery: a physiochemical and microbiologic evaluation of Merocel and NuGauze nasal packing. Laryngoscope 1987;97(12):1388–91.

12. Tom LW, Palasti S, Potsic WP, et al. The effects of gelatin film stents in the middle meatus. Am J Rhinol 1997;11(3):229–32.

13. Wee JH, Lee CH, Rhee CS, et al. Comparison between Gelfoam packing and no packing after endoscopic sinus surgery in the same patients. Eur Arch Otorhinolaryngol 2012;269(3):897–903.

14. Cho K-S, Park C-H, Hong S-L, et al. Comparative analysis of Cutanplast and Spongostan nasal packing after endoscopic sinus surgery: a prospective, randomized, multicenter study. Eur Arch Otorhinolaryngol 2015;272(7):1699–705.

15. Cho K-S, Shin S-K, Lee J-H, et al. The efficacy of Cutanplast nasal packing after endoscopic sinus surgery: a prospective, randomized, controlled trial. Laryngoscope 2013;123(3):564–8.

16. Jameson M, Gross CW, Kountakis SE. FloSeal use in endoscopic sinus surgery: effect on postoperative bleeding and synechiae formation. Am J Otolaryngol 2006;27(2):86–90.

17. Maccabee MS, Trune DR, Hwang PH. Effects of topically applied biomaterials on paranasal sinus mucosal healing. Am J Rhinol 2003;17(4):203–7.

18. Chandra RK, Conley DB, Kern RC. The effect of FloSeal on mucosal healing after endoscopic sinus surgery: a comparison with thrombin-soaked gelatin foam. Am J Rhinol 2003;17(1):51–5.

19. Chandra RK, Conley DB, Haines GK, et al. Long-term effects of FloSeal packing after endoscopic sinus surgery. Am J Rhinol 2005;19(3):240–3.

20. Miller RS, Steward DL, Tami TA, et al. The clinical effects of hyaluronic acid ester nasal dressing (Merogel) on intranasal wound healing after functional endoscopic sinus surgery. Otolaryngol Head Neck Surg 2003;128(6):862–9.

21. Franklin JH, Wright ED. Randomized, controlled, study of absorbable nasal packing on outcomes of surgical treatment of rhinosinusitis with polyposis. Am J Rhinol 2007;21(2):214–7.

22. Berlucchi M, Castelnuovo P, Vincenzi A, et al. Endoscopic outcomes of resorbable nasal packing after functional endoscopic sinus surgery: a multicenter prospective randomized controlled study. Eur Arch Otorhinolaryngol 2009;266(6):839–45.

23. Wormald PJ, Boustred RN, Le T, et al. A prospective single-blind randomized controlled study of use of hyaluronic acid nasal packs in patients after endoscopic sinus surgery. Am J Rhinol 2006;20(1):7–10.

24. Hu K-H, Lin K-N, Li W-T, et al. Effects of Meropack in the middle meatus after functional endoscopic sinus surgery in children with chronic sinusitis. Int J Pediatr Otorhinolaryngol 2008;72(10):1535–40.

25. Kimmelman CP, Edelstein DR, Cheng HJ. Sepragel sinus (hylan B) as a postsurgical dressing for endoscopic sinus surgery. Otolaryngol Head Neck Surg 2001; 125(6):603–8.

26. Frenkiel S, Desrosiers MY, Nachtigal D. Use of hylan B gel as a wound dressing after endoscopic sinus surgery. J Otolaryngol 2002;31(Suppl 1):S41–4.

27. Shi R, Zhou J, Wang B, et al. The clinical outcomes of new hyaluronan nasal dressing: a prospective, randomized, controlled study. Am J Rhinol Allergy 2013; 27(1):71–6.

28. Vaiman M, Eviatar E, Shlamkovich N, et al. Use of fibrin glue as a hemostatic in endoscopic sinus surgery. Ann Otol Rhinol Laryngol 2005;114(3):237–41.

29. Yu MS, Kang S-H, Kim B-H, et al. Effect of aerosolized fibrin sealant on hemostasis and wound healing after endoscopic sinus surgery: a prospective randomized study. Am J Rhinol Allergy 2014;28(4):335–40.

30. Erkan AN, Cakmak O, Kocer NE, et al. Effects of fibrin glue on nasal septal tissues. Laryngoscope 2007;117(3):491–6.

31. Al-Shaikh S, Muddaiah A, Lee RJ, et al. Oxidised cellulose powder for haemostasis following sinus surgery: a pilot randomised trial. J Laryngol Otol 2014;128(8): 709–13.

32. Kastl KG, Betz CS, Siedek V, et al. Control of bleeding following functional endoscopic sinus surgery using carboxy-methylated cellulose packing. Eur Arch Otorhinolaryngol 2009;266(8):1239–43.

33. Kastl KG, Betz CS, Siedek V, et al. Effect of carboxymethylcellulose nasal packing on wound healing after functional endoscopic sinus surgery. Am J Rhinol Allergy 2009;23(1):80–4.

34. Szczygielski K, Rapiejko P, Wojdas A, et al. Use of CMC foam sinus dressing in FESS. Eur Arch Otorhinolaryngol 2010;267(4):537–40.

35. Antisdel JL, Meyer A, Comer B, et al. Product comparison model in otolaryngology: equivalency analysis of absorbable hemostatic agents after endoscopic sinus surgery. Laryngoscope 2016;126(Suppl 2):S5–13.

36. Antisdel JL, West-Denning JL, Sindwani R. Effect of microporous polysaccharide hemospheres (MPH) on bleeding after endoscopic sinus surgery: randomized controlled study. Otolaryngol Head Neck Surg 2009;141(3):353–7.

37. Antisdel JL, Matijasec JL, Ting JY, et al. Microporous polysaccharide hemospheres do not increase synechiae after sinus surgery: randomized controlled study. Am J Rhinol Allergy 2011;25(4):268–71.

38. Beyea JA, Rotenberg BW. Comparison of purified plant polysaccharide (HemoStase) versus gelatin-thrombin matrix (FloSeal) in controlling bleeding during sinus surgery: a randomized controlled trial. Ann Otol Rhinol Laryngol 2011;120(8): 495–8.

39. Valentine R, Athanasiadis T, Moratti S, et al. The efficacy of a novel chitosan gel on hemostasis and wound healing after endoscopic sinus surgery. Am J Rhinol Allergy 2010;24(1):70–5.

40. Ngoc Ha T, Valentine R, Moratti S, et al. A blinded randomized controlled trial evaluating the efficacy of chitosan gel on ostial stenosis following endoscopic sinus surgery. Int Forum Allergy Rhinol 2013;3(7):573–80.

41. Shoman N, Gheriani H, Flamer D, et al. Prospective, double-blind, randomized trial evaluating patient satisfaction, bleeding, and wound healing using biodegradable synthetic polyurethane foam (NasoPore) as a middle meatal spacer in functional endoscopic sinus surgery. J Otolaryngol 2009;38(1):112–8.

42. Verim A, Seneldir L, Naiboğlu B, et al. Role of nasal packing in surgical outcome for chronic rhinosinusitis with polyposis. Laryngoscope 2014;124(7):1529–35.

43. Kastl KG, Reichert M, Scheithauer MO, et al. Patient comfort following FESS and Nasopore packing, a double blind, prospective, randomized trial. Rhinology 2014;52(1):60–5.

44. Song KJ, Lee HM, Lee EJ, et al. Anti-adhesive effect of a thermosensitive poloxamer applied after the removal of nasal packing in endoscopic sinus surgery: a randomised multicentre clinical trial. Clin Otolaryngol 2013;38(3):225–30.

45. Eliashar R, Gross M, Wohlgelernter J, et al. Packing in endoscopic sinus surgery: is it really required? Otolaryngol Head Neck Surg 2006;134(2):276–9.

46. Orlandi RR, Lanza DC. Is nasal packing necessary following endoscopic sinus surgery? Laryngoscope 2004;114(9):1541–4.

Trends in the Use of Stents and Drug-Eluting Stents in Sinus Surgery

Leah J. Hauser, MD, Justin H. Turner, MD, PhD,
Rakesh K. Chandra, MD*

KEYWORDS

- Sinus surgery • Chronic rhinosinusitis • Chronic sinusitis • Stents
- Drug-eluting stents • Steroid releasing stents

KEY POINTS

- Steroid-impregnated dressings and implants appear to be safe, although likely have increased systemic absorption compared with topical nasal steroid sprays and rinses.
- There is evidence to support the use of steroid-releasing implants in the ethmoid cavity; however, more study is needed to truly define the role of these implants.
- Slow resorbing steroid-releasing implants may be a promising option for the treatment of recurrent nasal polyposis in select patients.
- Maintaining patency of the frontal sinus outflow tract has unique challenges, where stenting and drug delivery may have benefit.

INTRODUCTION

The success rate of endoscopic sinus surgery (ESS) is high. However, a subset of patients has continued disease requiring further medical therapy and/or revision surgery.[1,2] Failures and suboptimal postoperative outcomes may be due to recurrent inflammatory disease, scarring/synechiae, ostial stenosis, or middle turbinate lateralization. Postoperative care, including steroids and middle meatal stents or spacers, can minimize some of these failures to optimize outcomes after sinus surgery.[3]

Stenting has long been used in the paranasal sinuses with the goals of maintaining a patent sinus cavity during the postoperative healing process and preventing restenosis from inflammation or scarring. Although the practice of stenting may be a mainstay in other settings of luminal surgery, use in ESS continues to evolve with scientific

Disclosure Statement: L.J. Hauser has nothing to disclose. J.H. Turner is a Consultant for IntersectENT. R.K. Chandra is a Consultant for Meda, J&J, Olympus, and IntersectENT.
Department of Otolaryngology, Division of Rhinology, Sinus & Skull Base Surgery, Vanderbilt University, 1215 21st Avenue South, #7209 MCE South Tower, Nashville, TN 37232-8605, USA
* Corresponding author.
E-mail address: Rakesh.Chandra@vanderbilt.edu

Otolaryngol Clin N Am 50 (2017) 565–571
http://dx.doi.org/10.1016/j.otc.2017.01.007
0030-6665/17/© 2017 Elsevier Inc. All rights reserved.

advances and clinical experience, and the exact indications for use of stents are still currently debated. Options include a wide array of both rigid and pliable absorbable and nonabsorbable materials. More recently, drug-eluting stents have been introduced and have been well studied.

Clinical experience supports the use of steroids postoperatively, although the ideal delivery system continues to be debated. Systemic steroids are very effective at decreasing postoperative edema and promoting healing postoperatively; however, there is the potential for significant side effects, including aseptic necrosis of the femoral head, uncontrolled hyperglycemia in diabetics, and orbital and psychiatric complications.[4] Topical steroid delivery systems have therefore been preferred when feasible. Nasal steroid sprays are safe and effective, but have limited penetration into the paranasal sinuses.[5] High-volume budesonide irrigations have been shown to be effective,[6] but possible concerns exist over the safety profile when these are used over extended periods, particularly with regard to hypothalamic-pituitary-adrenal suppression.[7,8] Recent trends have included targeted steroid placement, using topical steroid combined with existing (usually bioabsorbable) dressings, and also the application of manufactured drug-eluting stents engineered specifically to achieve this end. The present report focuses on materials that have been used for targeted steroid delivery, and stents specifically manufactured to achieve this purpose.

Steroid-Impregnated Dressings

Steroid impregnation of existing biomaterial dressings was a strategy developed to combine the potential advantages of stenting the middle turbinate medially with improved healing via controlled local drug delivery, with minimal systemic absorption.

Two randomized, double-blind, placebo controlled trials have evaluated steroid-impregnated dressings with conflicting results. Cote and Wright[9] studied 19 patients using a triamcinolone- versus saline-impregnated bioabsorbable proprietary polyurethane foam dressing (Nasopore; Stryker, Kalamazoo, MI, USA) and found statistically improved nasal endoscopy scores at 3 and 6 months after surgery in the triamcinolone group. Rudmik and colleagues[10] found no statistical difference in endoscopy scores among 36 patients in a randomized placebo controlled trial where the cavities in one arm were treated with dexamethasone-containing carboxyethyl cellulose foam (Stammberger Sinu-Foam; Smith & Nephew, London, UK), while the others received foam mixed with saline. It should be noted, however, that the study protocol included a course of oral steroids for all participants. More and colleagues[11] found that triamcinolone-impregnated matrix (Nasopore) was equivalent to a short course of oral steroids in combating the early return of edema in polyp patients, showing that steroid dressings can be used effectively outside the perioperative period.

Another study on safety of this triamcinolone-impregnated matrix (Nasopore) found a transient decrease in serum cortisol that normalized by postoperative day 10.[12] The investigators concluded that this change was likely not clinically significant, although the data imply that systemic steroid absorption from a saturated dressing may be higher than other topical steroid applications. A systematic review subsequently showed a trend toward decreased adhesions among steroid-impregnated versus placebo spacers, but data were unable to be pooled and analyzed given significant heterogeneity among studies.[13]

Manufactured Drug-Eluting Stents

A steroid-eluting stent composed of a polylactide-co-glycolide scaffold impregnated with 370 μg of mometasone furoate was designed by Intersect ENT (Propel, Menlo Park, CA, USA) in 2011 (**Fig. 1**).[14,15] It is meant to slowly release steroid by diffusion

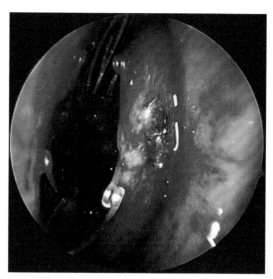

Fig. 1. Stent made of a polylactide-*co*-glycolide scaffold and impregnated with 370 μg of mometasone furoate. Stent deployed in a right ethmoid cavity.

in a controlled fashion over approximately 30 days.[14] Original testing in rabbits showed it to be safe with stable mucosal drug concentrations, minimal systemic absorption, and no significant inflammatory or ulcerative reactions.[15] The stents were nearly completely resorbed by 6 weeks, and no residual stent material was able to be detected at 18 weeks.

Safety and efficacy for use in humans were confirmed using a multicenter prospective randomized control.[14] A total of 38 subjects were included and served as their own controls, with a drug-eluting stent placed on one side and an identical nondrug stent placed on the control side. This study showed a statistically significant decrease in ethmoid sinus inflammation, polypoid change, adhesion formation, and middle turbinate lateralization in the treatment side versus the control side 3 to 6 weeks after surgery, but this effect did not persist 60 days after surgery.[14] Two multisite randomized double-blinded placebo control trials followed.[16,17] Forwith and colleagues[16] showed minimal rates of polyp formation, adhesions, and middle turbinate lateralization, with no changes in intraocular pressure, in 50 subjects treated with a steroid-containing stent compared with either a placebo stent on the contralateral side or controls from the Murr and colleagues[14] study. Marple and colleagues[17] further expanded on these results to show a 44.9% relative reduction in frank polyposis and a 61.6% relative reduction in significant adhesions at 30 days for the drug-eluting stent side compared with a placebo stent in 105 patients in an intrapatient design. There was also a 29.0% relative reduction in postoperative interventions, driven largely by the reduced number of lysis of adhesions performed, because there was no significant difference in need for oral steroids between the 2 groups.[17] A meta-analysis of pooled data from these randomized controlled trials that included 143 patients showed a 35% reduction in postoperative interventions ($P = .008$), including a decrease in lysis of adhesions by 51% ($P = .0016$) and 40% reduction in oral steroid use ($P = .0023$).[18]

Although generally well tolerated, stent misplacement, orbital injury, retained material, and chronic infection related to the stents have been reported.[19–21] US Food and Drug Administration (FDA) approval was granted in 2011 for use in the ethmoids postoperatively. Given these promising results, a *Cochrane Review* was undertaken in 2015 to evaluate the efficacy of drug-eluting stents compared with non-steroid-eluting stents, nasal packing, or no treatment. However, no conclusions were able to be drawn, as the intrapatient designs prevented the ability to perform health-related quality-of-life outcomes, and no studies were included.[22] The role of drug-eluting stents in the postoperative period continues to be a promising option, although it has been suggested that more studies are needed to show improved quality-of-life outcomes and to further define their role for patients with CRS without nasal polyposis.[3]

The mometasone-releasing stent was adapted for off-label in-office placement in patients with recurrence of polyps after ESS. The stent has a smaller arched profile and rounded tip for easier insertion in the awake patient and greater radial strength to dilate narrowed cavities and encourage stability in the ethmoid cavity during resolution of surrounding edema and polyps.[19,23,24] This new design was made with 1350 µg of mometasone furoate and engineered to resorb and elute the drug over 90 days, with most of the drug delivery in the first 30 days. A pilot study demonstrated feasibility of placement,[19] and a pharmacokinetic study showed no significant systemic absorption of steroid and no change in cortisol levels over the first 30 days.[23] A randomized controlled trial of 100 patients showed a significant reduction in polyps and a reduction in need for revision sinus surgery in patients receiving the treatment stent compared with a sham procedure at both 3 months[24] and 6 months.[25] With further study and FDA approval, this stent may be a good option to avoid revision surgery or repeated courses of oral steroids for patients with recurrent polyposis.

Stenting Considerations in the Frontal Sinus

The preceding discussion has largely focused on the role of stenting and drug delivery to maintain a patent middle meatus. With a narrow diameter and challenging anatomy, the frontal sinus is prone to narrowing and recurrent obstruction caused by inflammation and scar formation, and restenosis rates of up to 30% have been reported.[26] To combat this, along with meticulous dissection and advances in surgical technique, stenting is also commonly used in the frontal outflow tract. There are no widely accepted indications for placing frontal sinus stents, and routine stenting is not generally recommended given risks for obstruction of the stent in a narrow recess, granulation tissue formation, infection, and biofilm formation.[26] Stents have been suggested for circumferential bone exposure, extensive polyp disease or allergic fungal sinusitis, a flail or lateralized middle turbinate, and an intraoperative diameter of the frontal sinus ostium of less than 5 mm.[26,27] Although the percentage of patients in whom stents are used varies by surgeon preference, one skilled rhinologist reported using stents in 2.2% of his patients.[27] Others have used stents as an alternative to aggressive surgical intervention when medical comorbidities limit ability to undergo general anesthesia.[28] The ideal duration for stenting has also not been defined. Most investigators recommend at least 6 weeks, but reports of prolonged stenting for years have been published.[27,29] Many different materials have been used, including rigid metallic stents, and more recently, silicone or silastic sheeting or tubing and steroid-releasing implants.[30] Rains[31] described using a radiopaque, soft silicone tube with a collapsible bulb at one end in 67 patients, and this continues to be one of the most commonly used commercially available frontal sinus stents (**Fig. 2**).[27,28] More recently, in 2016, a modification of the previously discussed mometasone furoate–releasing bioabsorbable implant was FDA approved for use in the frontal sinus. In a randomized controlled trial of 67 patients, a 38.1% relative reduction in need for postoperative interventions after 30 days was seen for the treatment stent side compared with the surgery-alone side in an intrapatient design.[32] Stenosis of the

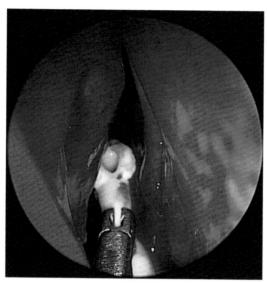

Fig. 2. Rains stent being placed in a right frontal sinus.

frontal sinus continues to be a challenging problem, and stenting is an option in select patients.

SUMMARY

Steroid-impregnated dressings and implants appear to be safe, although they likely have increased systemic absorption compared with topical nasal steroid sprays and rinses. There is evidence to support the use of steroid-releasing implants in the ethmoid cavity and frontal sinuses in the postoperative period; however, large trials have not been completed to show significant subjective and objective improvements over surgery alone with meticulous debridement and postoperative care. Slow resorbing steroid-releasing implants may be a promising option for the treatment of recurrent nasal polyposis in select patients. Maintaining patency of the frontal sinus outflow tract has unique challenges, where stenting and drug delivery may have benefit. Ultimately, the decision to use stents and steroid-releasing implants should be based on surgeon preference and clinical judgment. The role of these devices will likely continue to evolve with new innovations and changes in device approval.

REFERENCES

1. Senior BA, Kennedy DW, Tanabodee J, et al. Long-term results of functional endoscopic sinus surgery. Laryngoscope 1998;108:151–7.

2. Smith TL, Litvack JR, Hwang PH, et al. Determinants of outcomes of sinus surgery: a multi-institutional prospective cohort study. Otolaryngol Head Neck Surg 2010;142(1):55–63.

3. Rudmik L, Smith TL. Evidence-based practice: postoperative care in endoscopic sinus surgery. Otolaryngol Clin North Am 2012;45(5):1019–32.

4. Wright ED, Agrawal S. Impact of perioperative systemic steroids on surgical outcomes in patients with chronic rhinosinusitis with polyposis: evaluation with the

novel perioperative sinus endoscopy (POSE) scoring system. Laryngoscope 2007;117(11 pt 2 suppl 115):1–28.

5. Bonfils P, Nores JM, Halmi P, et al. Corticosteroid treatment in nasal polyposis with a three-year follow-up period. Laryngoscope 2003;113:683–7.

6. Snidvongs K, Pratt E, Chin D, et al. Corticosteroid nasal irrigations after endoscopic sinus surgery in the management of chronic rhinosinusitis. Int Forum Allergy Rhinol 2012;2(5):415–21.

7. Soudry E, Wang J, Vaezeafshar R, et al. Safety analysis of long-term budesonide nasal irrigations in patients with chronic rhinosinusitis post endoscopic sinus surgery. Int Forum Allergy Rhinol 2016;6:568–72.

8. Smith KA, French G, Mechor B, et al. Safety of long-term high-volume sinonasal budesonide irrigations for chronic rhinosinusitis. Int Forum Allergy Rhinol 2016;6: 228–32.

9. Cote DW, Wright ED. Triamcinolone-impregnated nasal dressing following endoscopic sinus surgery: a randomized, double-blind, placebo-controlled study. Laryngoscope 2010;120:1269–73.

10. Rudmik L, Mace J, Mechor B. Effect of a dexamethasone Sinu-Foam™ middle meatal spacer on endoscopic sinus surgery outcomes in patients with chronic rhinosinusitis without nasal polyposis: a randomized, double-blind, placebo-controlled trial. Int Forum Allergy Rhinol 2012;2:248–51.

11. More Y, Willen S, Catalano P. Management of early nasal polyposis using a steroid-impregnated nasal dressing. Int Forum Allergy Rhinol 2011;1(5):401–4.

12. Hong SD, Kim JH, Dhong HJ, et al. Systemic effects and safety of triamcinolone-impregnated nasal packing after endoscopic sinus surgery: a randomized, double-blinded, placebo-controlled study. Am J Rhinol Allergy 2013;27(5): 407–10.

13. Zhao X, Grewal A, Briel M, et al. A systematic review of nonabsorbable, absorbable, and steroid-impregnated spacers following endoscopic sinus surgery. Int Forum Allergy Rhinol 2013;3:896–904.

14. Murr AH, Smith TL, Hwang PH, et al. Safety and efficacy of a novel bioabsorbable, steroid-eluting sinus stent. Int Forum Allergy Rhinol 2011;1(1):23–32.

15. Li PM, Downie D, Hwang PH. Controlled steroid delivery via bioabsorbable stent: safety and performance in a rabbit model. Am J Rhinol Allergy 2009;23(6):591–6.

16. Forwith KD, Chandra RK, Yun PT, et al. ADVANCE: a multisite trial of bioabsorbable steroid-eluting sinus implants. Laryngoscope 2011;121(11):2473–80.

17. Marple BF, Smith TL, Han JK, et al. Advance II: a prospective, randomized study assessing safety and efficacy of bioabsorbable steroid-releasing sinus implants. Otolaryngol Head Neck Surg 2012;146(6):1004–11.

18. Han JK, Marple BF, Smith TL, et al. Effect of steroid releasing sinus implants on postoperative medical and surgical interventions: an efficacy meta-analysis. Int Forum Allergy Rhinol 2012;2:271–9.

19. Lavigne F, Miller SK, Gould AR, et al. Steroid-eluting sinus implant for in-office treatment of recurrent nasal polyposis: a prospective, multicenter study. Int Forum Allergy Rhinol 2014;4(5):381–9.

20. Kounis NG, Soufras GD, Hahalis G. Stent hypersensitivity and infection in sinus cavities. Allergy Rhinol (Providence) 2013;4(3):e162–5.

21. Vilari CR, Wojno TJ, Delgaudio JM. Case report of orbital violation with placement of ethmoid drug-eluting stent. Inf Forum Allergy Rhinol 2012;2(1):89–92.

22. Huang Z, Hwang P, Sun Y, et al. Steroid-eluting sinus stents for improving symptoms in chronic rhinosinusitis patients undergoing functional endoscopic sinus surgery. Cochrane Database Syst Rev 2015;(6):CD010436.

23. Ow R, Groppo E, Clutter D, et al. Steroid-eluting sinus implant for in-office treatment of recurrent polyposis: a pharmacokinetic study. Int Forum Allergy Rhinol 2014;4:816–22.
24. Han JK, Forwith SD, Smith TL, et al. RESOLVE: a randomized, controlled, blinded study of bioabsorbable steroid-eluting sinus implants for in-office treatment of recurrent sinonasal polyposis. Int Forum Allergy Rhinol 2014;4(11):861–70.
25. Forwith KD, Han JK, Stolovitzky JP, et al. RESOLVE: bioabsorbable steroid-eluting sinus implants for in-office treatment of recurrent sinonasal polyposis after sinus surgery: 6-month outcomes from a randomized, controlled, blinded study. Int Forum Allergy Rhinol 2016;6(6):573–81.
26. Kanowitz SJ, Jacobs JB, Lebowitz RA. "Frontal Sinus Stenting." The frontal sinus. In: Kountakis SE, Senior BA, Draf W, editors. Heidelberg (Germany): Springer; 2005. p. 261–6.
27. Orlandi RR, Knight J. Prolonged stenting of the frontal sinus. Laryngoscope 2009; 119(1):190–2.
28. Hunter B, Silva S, Youngs R, et al. Long-term stenting for chronic frontal sinus disease: case series and literature review. J Laryngol Otol 2010;124(11):1216–22.
29. Weber R, Mai R, Hosemann W, et al. The success of 6-month stenting in endonasal frontal sinus surgery. Ear Nose Throat J 2000;79(12):930–2.
30. Freeman SB, Blom ED. Frontal sinus stents. Laryngoscope 2000;110(7):1179–82.
31. Rains BM. Frontal sinus stenting. Otolaryngol Clin North Am 2001;34(1):101–10.
32. Smith TL, Singh A, Luong A, et al. Randomized controlled trial of a bioabsorbable steroid-releasing implant in the frontal sinus opening. Laryngoscope 2016; 126(12):2659–64.

Innovations in Balloon Catheter Technology in Rhinology

 CrossMark

Brian D'Anza, MD[a], Raj Sindwani, MD, FACS[b],
Troy D. Woodard, MD[b],*

KEYWORDS

- Balloon catheter technology • Balloon sinus dilation • Chronic sinus disease
- Endoscopic sinus surgery

KEY POINTS

- Balloon catheter technology (BCT) continues to expand as innovations in lighted guidewires, compatibility with surgical navigation, and ergonomics help to increase the scope of utilization.
- "Hybrid" balloon catheter dilation procedures are becoming more common, and there is high-quality literature supporting their use in improving outcomes.
- Indications for BCT have been bolstered by randomized controlled clinical trials showing durable improvement in quality of life and radiological outcomes in appropriately selected patients.
- Further prospective clinical trials are needed comparing stand-alone BCT with traditional endoscopic sinus surgery to help determine the specific patient populations that would benefit.

INTRODUCTION

The use of balloon catheter technology (BCT) is one of the more recent advances in the treatment of chronic rhinosinusitis (CRS). In 2015, the US market exploded, and the fastest growing segment of ear, nose, throat (ENT) endoscopic devices was balloon technologies.[1] Fueled by the demand for minimally invasive technologies and expanded insurance coverage, the marketplace for BCT was estimated to increase in value from approximately $50 million in 2012 to more than $200 million in 2015.

[a] Section of Rhinology and Skull Base Surgery, Department of Otolaryngology, University Hospitals–Case Western Reserve University, 11100 Euclid Avenue, Cleveland, OH 44106, USA;
[b] Section of Rhinology and Skull Base Surgery, Minimally Invasive Cranial Base & Pituitary Surgery Program, Head and Neck Institute, Burkhardt Brain Tumor and Neuro-Oncology Center, Cleveland Clinic Foundation, 9500 Euclid Avenue #A-71, Cleveland, OH 44195, USA
* Corresponding author.
E-mail address: woodart@ccf.org

Otolaryngol Clin N Am 50 (2017) 573–582
http://dx.doi.org/10.1016/j.otc.2017.01.008

The technology was first introduced as a treatment of chronic sinusitis in 2005 with US Food and Drug Administration approval of the Balloon Sinuplasty device (Acclarent, Inc, Menlo Park, CA, USA).

BCT has been present in other fields within medicine for decades. It was not until the early twenty-first century that experiments began with its use in dilating sinus ostia.[2,3] The initial devices were modifications of cardiac stenting balloons that provided a non-conforming balloon appliance fed over a flexible guidewire.[2]

Over the last 10 years, there have been many innovations in BCT as a therapy for paranasal sinus disease. The devices now permit multisinus applications using just one device and are equipped with suction and irrigation capabilities. They have also improved in ergonomics, and the methods of localization have expanded. Initial BCT localization was via fluoroscopy with the inherent risks of exposure to radiation. Today, recent advances include the utilization of transillumination and real-time 3-dimensional image guidance. The goals of this article are to explore these innovations and focus on the specific details of the technologies and utilities involved. This comprehensive review also examines the indications and limitations of BCT as evidenced in the contemporary literature.

INNOVATIONS IN SPECIFIC BALLOON CATHETER TECHNOLOGIES

BCTs have seen many generations developed from several companies over the years. They were initially conceived in the early portion of the twenty-first century as a distinct minimally invasive procedure that could serve as another tool in the treatment of CRS. In 2004, Acclarent Inc was the first company to begin development of BCT in treatment of sinus disease.[4] Multiple US patents have been obtained on the system, which uses a guidewire over which a sheath is passed to introduce the balloon into the targeted sinus (**Fig. 1**).

Entellus Medical, Inc (Maple Grove, MN, USA) was founded in 2006 as a company developing sinus-specific balloon technology. Their initial product was the Functional Infundibular Endoscopic Sinus System that proceeded through a transantral route. In 2010, Entellus developed a device using a transnasal route for dilation, irrigation, and suctioning of the frontal, sphenoid, or maxillary sinus ostia. It functions by using a flexible and malleable distal cannula along with an overlying balloon catheter to directly palpate and cannulate an ostium (**Fig. 2**). The more invasive transantral technique of approaching the maxillary sinus ostium from inside out via canine puncture has been largely abandoned.

More recently, Medtronic Inc (Minneapolis, MN, USA) has become involved in BCT with the release of their balloon platform, which can be readily coupled with their (EM) surgical navigation system. In 2014, Medtronic began offering a product called the NuVent EM Balloon sinus dilation system (**Fig. 3**), which offers a "plug and play" ability to track the tip of the balloon instrument obviating calibration.

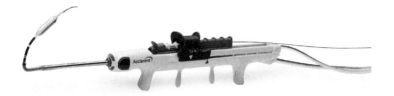

Fig. 1. Acclarent Relieva spin plus balloon sinuplasty system. (*Courtesy of* Acclarent Inc, Menlo Park, CA; with permission.)

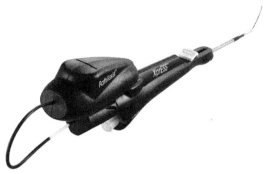

Fig. 2. Entellus XprESS ultra balloon dilation system. (*Courtesy of* Entellus Inc, Plymouth, MN.)

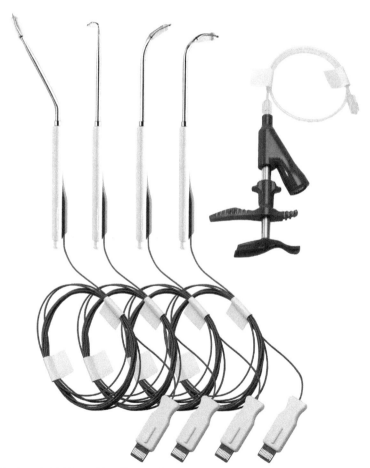

Fig. 3. Medtronic NuVent EM Balloon Dilation System including various angled seekers for access to multiple sinuses. (*Reprinted with the permission of* Medtronic, Inc. © 2016.)

Current BCT dilates a balloon over a flexible guidewire platform or over a rigid or semirigid probelike instrument. In the following sections, the most innovative design features pertaining to each of these platforms are explored.

Lighted Guidewire Localization Systems

Navigation of the balloon catheters initially relied on fluoroscopic guidance or direct visualization for appropriate placement. Recently, there has been a focus on lighted guidewire systems. The systems operate by cannulating the sinus openings in an atraumatic fashion and use a light-emitting diode (LED) light system. Once the target sinus is cannulated and entered, it is transilluminated with the LED on the end of the lighted guidewire. The focal intensity of the light and its movement when the lighted guidewire is "spun" or manipulated provides visual confirmation of correct positioning within the sinus interior. Transillumination confirms correct placement, and the balloon catheter can be deployed overtop of the guidewire using the Seldinger technique, allowing for accurate and direct treatment of the outflow obstruction. Compared with the prior fluoroscopic guidance, these devices are easier to implement and do not require exposure of the patient or operator to radiation.

The 2 most popular versions of this platform include the Acclarent Luma Sinus Illumination system (**Fig. 4**) and the Entellus PathAssist LED Light Fiber. Both of these devices can be used to allow for illumination of the affected sinus or sinuses, but function in different ways. The Entellus device permits localization with a short flexible guidewire for localization with balloon dilation remaining on the rigid cannula. Meanwhile, the Acclarent devices are able to dilate the balloon more distally along the flexible guidewire. Ballooning on the extended wire offers the advantage of "greater reach," into the frontal sinus for example, whereby even intrafrontal sinus obstruction (such as a type 3 frontal cell) can be managed. The Acclarent device has an adaptor that allows it to connect to most intraoperative lighting systems to improve ease of use. The

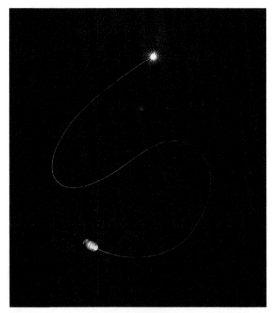

Fig. 4. Acclarent Luma Sinus Illumination system showing the lighted guidewire used for navigation. (*Courtesy of* Acclarent Inc, Menlo Park, CA; with permission.)

Entellus device light can be powered via an attached battery pack, eliminating the need for an additional power source and attendant cables.

Image-guided Balloon Catheter Technologies

The NuVent EM Balloon dilation system relies on Medtronic's intraoperative EM imaging technology called the Fusion ENT navigation system. The innovative design provides for balloon dilation devices that are precalibrated at the factory to match with the Fusion system. The BCT is meant for single use and has built-in AxiEM tracking abilities when paired with the Fusion system. The system is different than other BCTs in that the devices are all rigid with no malleable or flexible parts. The Rigidity is imperative to the function of the system because it relies entirely on the EM tracking abilities to ensure correct placement. The Rigidity allows for "plug and play" functionality because the devices are ready to use and track real time. There is no need for additional power sources, lights, or cords.

In addition, the Acclarent and Entellus devices also have image-guided functionalities with certain versions of their devices. The Relieva Scout Sinus dilation system (Acclarent, Inc) offers the option for navigation capabilities when used with optical-based navigation systems such as the BrainLab (Feldkirchen, Germany) Kolibri system. Meanwhile, the Entellus devices are compatible with intraoperative image guidance via the Fiagon Navigation System.

Other Innovations in Balloon Catheter Technology Construction

Some recent advances include improved ergonomics and functionality. Some newer Acclarent devices allow for integration of irrigation into the distal tip of the balloon without the need to remove the balloon or change the setup. Many of these newer devices provide cannula tips that are softer, narrower, and more flexible, helping minimize trauma to surrounding tissues. Just as important, several systems now limit the amount of attachments or add-ons required to approach multiple sinuses. The Acclarent devices all have built-in irrigation tips at the end of the cannulas, allowing irrigation and suctioning. Entellus devices have a malleable tip allowing for the utilization of one device for multiple sinuses without the need to change tips at all.

Innovations in Utilization of Balloon Catheter Technology

Traditional endoscopic sinus surgery (ESS) has typically been performed under general anesthesia. Standard techniques have long been described that revolve around opening large pathways via dissection and removal of diseased sinus air cells. BCT offers an alternative, advertised as a minimally invasive approach that is mucosal sparing, and with limited pain and convalescence. However, most initial reports of BCT usage were in the operating room under general anesthesia,[5,6] even though prospects were always enticing for balloon dilations to be performed on awake patients in the office. After the initial introduction, some physicians began offering BCT as a stand-alone alternative to ESS. Patient demand for the procedure was based partially on the convenience of avoiding general anesthesia and the requisite recovery time this entailed. Over the last several years, in-office use of the device has become commonplace. There is growing acceptance of BCT as an alternative way to treat certain types of sinus disease. In fact, a recent survey of the American Rhinologic Society (ARS) revealed that most members do use BCT in their practices and thought their usage of it in the coming years was likely to increase.[7]

In 2012, Albritton and colleagues[8] published data known as the ORIOS-1 study: a prospective, multicenter, nonrandomized trial evaluating the feasibility and safety of BCT utilization in an office-based setting under local anesthesia. Successful in-office balloon dilation of various sinuses was performed in 33 of 37 patients. The investigators reported statistically and clinically significant improvements in SNOT-20 scores and Lund-McKay Scores (LMK) after 1 year. ORIOS-1 was followed up with a larger sample size with similar design in the ORIOS-2 study.[9] In this trial, 93.2% of 532 patients had successful cannulation of various sinuses. Significant reductions in SNOT-20 and LMK were maintained and patient satisfaction remained high, with nearly three-quarters reporting they would have the procedure again. As well, the average time for return to work was 2.2 days, highlighting the benefits of BCT utilization in an ambulatory setting.

Since the inception of BCT in sinus treatment, innovations in so-called hybrid procedures have become popular. "Hybrid" procedures refer to when BCT is used as an adjunct to other instruments in performing ESS, typically in the operating room setting. In 2015, Hathorn and colleagues[10] reported a single-blinded, controlled, prospective cohort study using BCT in a hybrid approach to opening the frontal sinus ostium. All patients had initial exposure of the frontal recess via standard instrumentation. They then had frontal sinusotomy via a Draf 2A approach using standard instruments on one side, followed by balloon dilation of the contralateral side. They reported equivalence between the 2 techniques as all 30 frontal sinus ostia were successfully opened. All assessed ostia were patent at 3-month and 1-year follow-up. They noted hybrid balloon dilation decreased the average surgical time by nearly 5 minutes ($P = .03$). The results led the investigators to conclude the hybrid balloon technique to be a viable alternative to traditional frontal sinusotomy with equivalent short-term patency outcomes.

Brodner and colleagues[11] reported on outcomes of a subset of 175 patients who underwent hybrid-balloon procedures involving maxillary, frontal, and sphenoid sinuses. They found that of the 44 patients who completed 1-year follow-up there was significant improvement in average symptom scores from 1.9 to 0.8 ($P = .00001$). They reported the need for only one revision surgery.

These studies are representative of the growing evidence showing the benefits of hybrid utilization of BCT. It provides another tool to assist the surgeon in opening narrow ostia and drainage pathways while preserving mucosa. BCT clearly appears to have a role in the future direction of some forms of CRS.

INDICATIONS AND LIMITATIONS

In December 2012, the American Academy of Otolaryngology–Head and Neck Surgery (AAO-HNS) reaffirmed its position statement on "Balloon Sinus Ostial Dilation." In the statement, the Academy supported the use of a balloon as an "appropriate therapeutic option" in the treatment of sinusitis in "select" patients.[12] The final decision regarding use of a balloon was left to the discretion of the attending surgeon. It reaffirmed this statement in 2012, and in 2015, the ARS released its own position statement on balloon dilation, which echoed the AAO-HNS.[13] Since this time, several large insurance companies have adopted BCT as a therapeutic option for CRS that is reimbursable. United HealthCare, one of the largest insurers in the country, released a revised medical policy statement in February 2016 regarding "Balloon Sinus Ostial Dilation."[14] In this statement, the use of BCT was described as "medically necessary" if the following criteria are met:

1. CRS of the affected sinus is confirmed by computed tomographic scan findings of at least one of the following: mucosal thickening, bony remodeling, bony thickening, or obstruction of the ostiomeatal complex.
2. Balloon sinus ostial dilation is limited to the frontal, maxillary, or sphenoid sinuses.

3. Balloon sinus ostial dilation is performed stand-alone or in combination with standard FESS.
4. Patient must be 12 years of age or older.
5. Failure of medical therapy including: nasal lavage, antibiotic therapy (if bacterial infection is suspected), and topical corticosteroid use.

Despite the acceptance of BCT as a viable and safe option in the treatment of CRS, there have been controversies regarding the exact role and who qualifies as a "select patient." Not surprisingly, the addition of this new technology has created activists and opponents alike. Literature has focused on the benefits in symptom scores and objective criteria often found in large retrospective database reviews or prospective, single-armed trials.[15–19] Many of these results show functional benefits of BCT, with some even arguing for equivalency between balloon dilation and traditional ESS.[20] Initial reports displayed promise for BCT but had limitations in retrospective design, lack of control arms, relatively short follow-up times, or stringent inclusion criteria.[4,5,15–19]

One of the first prospective, longitudinal studies to be released with evidence of the benefits of BCT was the CLEAR study.[4,5,21] Results of this study were published in a series of 3 articles comparing preoperative and postoperative outcomes at 6-, 12-, and 24-month follow-up times. Statistically significant improvements in SNOT-20 and LMK scores were noted across all the studies and maintained through 24 months. The main issues raised with this study were the lack of a control arm and no randomization. Critics regarded these shortfalls as evidence that the benefits of BCT were not applicable to many patient populations. As a result, several randomized clinical trials, meta-analyses, and other prospective data have been published over the last 5 to 6 years.[22–24] These new studies have contributed to the discussion regarding the indications and limitations of BCT.

In 2013, Cutler and colleagues[25] published the first of 2 parts of the REMODEL study (Randomized Evaluation of Maxillary antrostomy vs Ostial Dilation Efficacy through Long-term follow-up). This study was the first randomized, controlled, clinical trial of sufficient statistical power comparing stand-alone BCT to traditional ESS. It used Entellus BCT and enrolled a total of 105 patients who were randomized to either the control ESS arm or the experimental BCT arm. In total, 42 ESS-treated patients and 49 BCT-treated patients completed the 6-month follow-up. Significant improvements in SNOT-20 scores were seen in both the BCT and the ESS arms. The investigators concluded there was evidence for "noninferiority" between BCT and ESS. The inclusion criteria were stringent, however, and only maxillary sinuses were treated with dilation. In addition, patients were excluded if they had posterior ethmoid, frontal, or sphenoid sinus disease. Patients with gross polypoid disease, fungal disease, severe septal deviation, and comorbidities, such as aspirin-exacerbated respiratory disease (AERD) and hemophilia, were excluded.

In 2014, Bikhazi and colleagues[26] released the second part of the REMODEL study, which included longer-term follow-up results over 12 months. They found that the SNOT-20 score improvements were durable over this time period as were most of the secondary outcome measures mentioned above. Then, Chandra and colleagues[27] reported on the final outcomes of the REMODEL trial, including a larger cohort of 135 patients with longer-term follow-up. In addition, they performed a meta-analysis of 6 studies in the literature reviewing stand-alone BCT versus FESS. They found that 2-year SNOT-20 outcomes of the REMODEL trial were similar to those found in the meta-analysis. They concluded that outcomes are comparable to the 6-month time points in the initial REMODEL report. The Study was reported as evidence of significant, durable benefit in patients with limited maxillary sinus disease undergoing balloon dilation.

The literature is not without critics of BCT, because much of the randomized controlled clinical trials mentioned above have strict inclusion criteria and largely reflect patients with limited disease. As well, there are questions regarding the benefits of BCT in an era where cost containment and efficiency are becoming more important. In 2015, Ference and colleagues[27] published a retrospective cross-sectional analysis reviewing the utilization of BCT compared with traditional ESS. They used Current Procedural Terminology codes in State Ambulatory Surgery Databases for California, Florida, Maryland, and New York in 2011. A total of 33,776 patients were included. They found the median charges involving BCT to be nearly double that of traditional ESS ($4500 BCT vs $2950 ESS, $P = .003$). The median operating room time was statistically equivalent. This study offers pause for concern as BCT, as with any technology, may increase the burden of cost while not making a significant difference in operating time.

One of the most comprehensive recent studies looking at BCT is by Levy and colleagues.[28] This study, published in 2015, is a systematic review and meta-analysis of the MEDLINE and EMBASE databases. Studies were included when primary outcomes included the impact of BCT on validated measures of quality of life and sinus opacification. A total of 17 studies were included, all being either level 1 or 2 evidence. They found that BCT did show a statistically significant improvement in paranasal sinus opacification and SNOT-20 scores following balloon dilation. They only found 2 studies, however, that directly compared validated outcome measures between BCT and traditional ESS.[22,29] These studies did not demonstrate a significant difference in outcome. They concluded that current evidence regarding the role of BCT in CRS is limited. Long-term quality of life and radiographic improvements are seen in a "restricted" adult population with CRS. Clearly, further study is needed in specific subgroups and settings. As well, patients with certain diseases are nearly always excluded from randomized studies including fungal sinusitis, severe nasal polyposis, AERD, neoplasms, and severe septal deviation. Thus, there is no current evidence to support the use of BCT in these circumstances.

In the end, BCT has shown great promise, and there is high-quality evidence supporting its role in specific circumstances. Taking into account the above studies, BCT appears to currently have significant level 1 or 2 evidence supporting its use in maxillary and frontal sinuses in adult CRS patients without nasal polyposis. As well, the patient populations appear to have disease isolated to a single sinus, with evidence being greatest for treating maxillary and frontal sinus disease. There are, however, many within the field that think the role of stand-alone BCT exists in a wider context, such as with recurrent acute sinusitis, facial pain symptoms, and even polyp disease. Further study is needed to validate these indications and add clarity to the beneficial scope of BCT. As with any tool, effective usage hinges on a thorough understanding of how the instrument works, its limitations, and when it should and should not be used.

SUMMARY

BCT has undergone several generations of improvement since being first developed more than 10 years ago. There have been a myriad of updates and innovations to all aspects of BCT, from how devices are constructed, to how they are used, and the evidence to support them. The ergonomics of the balloon dilation systems have improved significantly with a focus on limiting the amount of setup for each device and simplifying their overall functioning. Studies have shown the benefits of hybrid balloon dilation procedures in treating isolated complex frontal disease. There is high-quality evidence showing the durable benefits of stand-alone BCT in treating patients with limited CRS. Multiple randomized, prospective clinical trials report improved long-term outcomes in BCT. Nearly all studies profile BCT being extremely safe and well tolerated, with a low complication rate. In certain circumstances, there is evidence to show it is equivalent to (limited) traditional ESS; however, further studies are needed. The ever-expanding technological innovations in BCT and evidence-based evaluations of their utility ensure these devices are a key component in the armamentarium of the contemporary sinus surgeon. Future study will better clarify indications for when this BCT can add value in the care of our sinus patients.

REFERENCES

1. Available at: http://idataresearch.com/. Accessed June 1, 2016.
2. Bolger WE, Vaughan WC. Catheter-based dilation of the sinus ostia: initial safety and feasibility analysis in a cadaver model. Am J Rhinol 2006;20:290–4.
3. Vaughan WC. Review of balloon sinuplasty. Curr Opin Otolaryngol Head Neck Surg 2008;16:2–9.
4. Batra PS, Ryan MW, Sindwani R, et al. Balloon catheter technology in rhinology: reviewing the evidence. Laryngoscope 2011;121(1):226–32.
5. Kuhn FA, Church CA, Goldberg AN, et al. Balloon catheter sinusotomy: one-year follow-up—outcomes and role in functional endoscopic sinus surgery. Otolaryngol Head Neck Surg 2008;139:S27–37.
6. Weiss RL, Church CA, Kuhn FA, et al. Long-term outcome analysis of balloon catheter sinusotomy: two-year follow-up. Otolaryngol Head Neck Surg 2008; 139:S38–46.
7. Halderman AA, Stokken J, Momin SR, et al. Attitudes on and usage of balloon catheter technology in rhinology: a survey of the American Rhinologic Society. Am J Rhinol Allergy 2015;29(5):389–93.
8. Albritton FDT, Casiano RR, Sillers MJ. Feasibility of in-office endoscopic sinus surgery with balloon sinus dilation. Am J Rhinol Allergy 2012;26:243–8.
9. Karanfilov B, Silvers S, Pasha R, et al. Office-based balloon sinus dilation: a prospective, multicenter study of 203 patients. Int Forum Allergy Rhinol 2013;3: 404–11.
10. Hathorn IF, Pace-Asciak P, Habib AR, et al. Randomized controlled trial: hybrid technique using balloon dilation of the frontal sinus drainage pathway. Int Forum Allergy Rhinol 2015;5(2):167–73.
11. Brodner D, Nachlas N, Mock P, et al. Safety and outcomes following hybrid balloon and balloon-only procedures using a multifunction, multisinus balloon dilation tool. Int Forum Allergy Rhinol 2013;3(8):652–8.
12. ENTnet.org. AAO-HNS Statement on Reimbursement of Balloon Sinus Ostial Dilation. 2014. Available at: http://www.entnet.org/content/position-statement-dilation-sinuses-any-method-eg-balloon-etc. Accessed June 5, 2016.
13. American-rhinologic.org. Ostial Balloon Dilation Position Statement. 2016. Available at: https://www.american-rhinologic.org/position_balloon_dilation. Accessed June 5, 2016.
14. 501(k) summary, Acclarent Inc. HHS provided. Available at: https://www.accessdata.fda.gov/cdrh_docs/pdf14/K143541.pdf. Accessed June 1, 2016.
15. Levine H, Sertich AP, Hoisington DR, et al. Multicenter registry of balloon catheter sinusotomy outcomes for 1036 patients. Ann Otol Rhinol Laryngol 2008;117(4): 265–70.

16. Friedman A, Schalch P, Lin SC, et al. Functional endoscopic dilatation of the sinuses: patient satisfaction, postoperative pain, and cost. Am J Rhinol 2008;22:204–9.
17. Levine SB, Truitt T, Schwartz M, et al. In-office stand-alone balloon dilation of maxillary sinus ostia and ethmoid infundibula in adults with chronic or recurrent acute rhinosinusitis: a prospective, multi-institutional study with-1-year follow-up. Ann Otol Rhinol Laryngol 2013;122(11):665–71.
18. Catalano PJ, Payne SC. Balloon dilation of the frontal recess in patients with chronic frontal sinusitis and advanced sinus disease: an initial report. Ann Otol Rhinol Laryngol 2009;118:107–12.
19. Friedman M, Wilson M. Illumination guided balloon sinuplasty. Laryngoscope 2009;119:1399–402.
20. Catalano PJ. Balloon dilation technology: let the truth be told. Curr Allergy Asthma Rep 2013;13:250–4.
21. Bolger WE, Brown CL, Church CA, et al. Safety and outcomes of balloon catheter sinusotomy: a multicenter 24-week analysis in 115 patients. Otolaryngol Head Neck Surg 2007;137:10–20.
22. Chandra RK, Kern RC, Cutler JL, et al. REMODEL larger cohort with long-term outcomes and meta-analysis of standalone balloon dilation studies. Laryngoscope 2016;126(1):44–50.
23. Browning GG. Updating a Cochrane review of endoscopic balloon dilation for chronic rhinosinusitis: a randomised controlled trial that is biased in its reporting. Clin Otolaryngol 2012;37(3):222.
24. Lefevre F, Rosenberg AB. Balloon dilation of the frontal recess: a randomized clinical trial. Ann Otol Rhinol Laryngol 2012;121(10):700 [author reply 700].
25. Cutler J, Bikhazi N, Light J, et al. Standalone balloon dilation versus sinus surgery for chronic rhinosinusitis: a prospective, multicenter, randomized, controlled trial. Am J Rhinol Allergy 2013;27:416–22.
26. Bikhazi N, Light J, Truitt T, et al. Standalone balloon dilation versus sinus surgery for chronic rhinosinusitis: a prospective, multicenter, randomized, controlled trial with 1-year followup. Am J Rhinol Allergy 2014;28:323–9.
27. Ference E, Graber M, Conley D, et al. Operative utilization of balloon versus traditional endoscopic sinus surgery. Laryngoscope 2015;125(1):49–56.
28. Levy JM, Marino MJ, McCoul ED. Paranasal sinus balloon catheter dilation for treatment of chronic rhinosinusitis: a systematic review and meta-analysis. Otolaryngol Head Neck Surg 2016;154(1):33–40.
29. Achar P, Duvvi S, Kumar BN. Endoscopic dilatation sinus surgery (FEDS) versus functional endoscopic sinus surgery (FESS) for treatment of chronic rhinosinusitis: a pilot study. Acta Otorhinolaryngol Ital 2012;32:314–9.

The Emerging Role of 3-Dimensional Printing in Rhinology

Janalee K. Stokken, MD*, John F. Pallanch, MD, MS

KEYWORDS

- Nasal septal perforation • Prosthetic closure • 3D printing • Computed tomography
- Septal prostheses

KEY POINTS

- The most common symptoms of nasal septal perforation are crusting, bleeding, difficulty breathing, pain, and rhinorrhea.
- Septal perforations larger than 2 cm can be difficult to surgically close and have a higher rate of reperforation than smaller defects.
- Three-dimensional (3D) printing technology offers a new technique for sizing custom septal buttons with a better fit than previously described methods.
- Patient retention rates are 90% when the 3D sizing method is used; symptom improvement rates are comparable with other techniques for septal perforation closure.

INTRODUCTION

The increasing availability of 3-dimensional (3D) printing has led to multiple applications in rhinology. These applications include the creation of accurate patient-specific preoperative models for procedure planning, rehearsal, and patient consultation. It allows for the production of patient-specific customized prostheses for multiple applications, including nasal septal perforations.

The anatomically accurate 3D printed models can be used before complex surgical cases to provide the surgeon with additional information on the location and orientation of a lesion. Modern 3D printers can print models of patients' unique anatomy and in multiple color components. This ability allows different structures within the model to be represented by different colors, demonstrating the difference between bone, soft tissue, tumor, or major vascular structures. Simulated surgery can be conducted on these models to plan osteotomies, better understand anatomic variants, practice

There are no conflicts of interest for either of the authors.
Department of Otorhinolaryngology, Mayo Clinic, 200 First Street SW, Rochester, MN 55905, USA
* Corresponding author:
E-mail address: stokken.janalee@mayo.edu

drilling near vital structures, or to develop templates for prostheses or reconstructive plates. These models provide the surgeon with conceptualization beyond what 3D image analysis offers. Models can also be printed with the removed to assist with reconstruction planning or to design a template for the future skull base defect.

Although most of the applications described earlier are used for complex skull base cases in tertiary care settings, 3D printing has a role in the general otolaryngologist's practice as well. Three-dimensional models can be used to create templates for maxillofacial trauma surgery or to design prosthetic implants. Prostheses can be designed for large and irregular septal perforations or defects caused by trauma or tumor ablation. This article discusses and provides examples of how 3D printing is improving the treatment of large or irregular nasal septal perforations by using both simulated surgery and prosthetic design.

Nasal septal perforations result from various causes, including previous nasal surgery, external nasal trauma, intranasal trauma, cocaine use, history of nasal cautery, and vasculitis.[1] Septal perforations can cause symptoms that range from minimal to severe, and they can significantly impact patients' quality of life. The most common symptoms are crusting, epistaxis, difficulty breathing, pain, rhinorrhea, postnasal drainage, hyposmia, malodor, and whistling.[1] Treatment options are tailored to the individual based on the severity of symptoms and size of the perforation. Nasal moisturizing agents are typically used as a first-line therapy and may be adequate therapy for the minimally symptomatic. Various surgical and nonsurgical closures have been used for more than 60 years in patients who do not respond to conservative topical agents.[2]

Surgical closure is a good option for small- to medium-sized defects, but successful closure can be difficult to attain for large and/or irregular perforations. A review of surgical methods for closure of septal perforation from 1960 to 2011 found that larger perforations (>2.0 cm) have a lower rate (73.8%) of successful surgical closure than smaller perforations.[3] Another review found a reperforation rate of 48% and attributed the failures to larger-sized perforations with unilateral mucosal closure.[4] The amount of available, nonscared mucosa relative to the size of the perforation is an important consideration. Since 1972, symptomatic patients with large nasal septal perforations, who were not candidates for surgery, have had the option of custom prosthetic closure at the Mayo Clinic.[5–7] Although septal prostheses have helped many patients, 27% of patients before 1982 chose not to keep the prosthesis in place because of discomfort.[8]

Before the 1980s, a custom prosthesis carved by a medical artist proved to be more comfortable than commercially available prostheses for large and irregular perforations. As accurate sizing remained a challenge, the carving technique was improved with the use of 2-dimensional (2D) computed tomography (CT) sizing[1,8]; more patients choose to keep their prosthesis. The introduction of 3D printing to the sizing process in 2007 offered the potential for further improvement by allowing the prosthesis to fit each patient's nasal anatomy exactly. The resulting product would provide more patient comfort and, thus, a higher retention rate. This article reviews how 3D printing technology is improving the fabrication of nasal septal prostheses for sizing nasal septal perforations.

EXPLANATION OF THE TECHNOLOGY
Image Data Acquisition and Printing

After patients are evaluated by an otolaryngologist, are not surgical candidates, and are found to be candidates for a septal prosthesis, a high-resolution CT of the face and paranasal sinuses is obtained (**Fig. 1**). The target resolution of the CT imaging

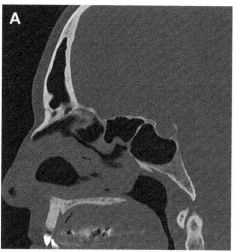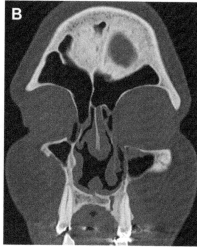

Fig. 1. (*A*) Sagittal and (*B*) coronal CT images of a patient with a large perforation. The coronal view highlights the thickened superior margin. The image set containing these images were used for sizing the prosthesis for this patient.

is between 0.29 and 0.49 mm isotropic resolution, and the slice thickness is less than 1 mm. The image data are then segmented and used to create a virtual 3D model of the perforated septum and surrounding tissue and the model is printed. The prosthetics department then creates the prosthesis using the printed 3D template.

Modifying the 3-Dimensional Printed Model

The additional step of simulated surgery can be taken before the prosthesis fabrication. This step is considered in cases whereby there are significant adhesions between the edges of the perforation and the lateral wall or there is extreme posterior septal thickening or obstructive bony remodeling that will be addressed at the time of button placement. The surgeon uses the model to perform a simulated surgery and create the desirable posterior and superior margins. These steps are then replicated at the time of surgery before placing the custom button. Printing the 3D templates in 2 colors, one for soft tissue and another for bone, will assist the surgeon in avoiding trauma to the skull base. The desired 3D model is then ready for fabrication of the prosthesis.

Prosthesis Fabrication

The 3D model is then trimmed to expose the margins of the septal perforation. The trimmed 3D model is duplicated using a technique that is similar to the technique used to create custom dental (whitening) trays. A dental impression material is placed over the model, which is then used to make a stone cast that can withstand the heat and pressure needed to make the polymeric silicone prosthesis. The Lost Wax technique is used; a molding wax is pressed into the casted model in the shape of the future prosthesis, ensuring an exact fit. The edges of the prosthesis are tapered and minimized to decrease the risk of nasal airway obstruction. Another cast of dental stone is created over the wax to form a 2-piece mold. The wax is removed from the mold using boiling water, which creates a space for crafting the actual patient prosthesis. Lastly, the mold is filled with medical-grade polymeric silicone, placed in a press, and left overnight in a dry-heat oven at 120°F. The entire process typically takes about a week to complete.

INDICATIONS

A custom prosthesis can be placed in any symptomatic perforation but is ideal for perforations that are large (>1.5 cm) and difficult to surgically close (**Fig. 2**). The authors have also found that patients who have not tolerated commercially available buttons previously can be successfully closed with a custom prosthesis. A 3D-sized custom button can be considered in patients who are poor candidates for a general anesthetic, who are taking anticoagulation, with active granulomatous or vascular disease, or who just cannot tolerate surgery or the perioperative requirements, for example, postoperative splinting for 2 weeks.

Placement of the Prosthesis

Once the polymeric silicone prosthesis is complete, it is delivered, along with the casted stone model, to the surgeon. The button can be placed in the operating room or in a clinic procedure room. Some prostheses are easier to place and are well tolerated by patients, with only topical anesthesia. An operative setting would be desired if the prosthesis is much larger than the nares opening, if there is planned concomitant lysis of adhesions or trimming of bone (as described in the cases in which the patient's model had simulated surgery as part of the design), or if sinus surgery is required.

The prosthesis is rinsed in a sterilizing solution, and then 1 or 2 sutures[9] are placed to bend the left superior and inferior flanges toward each other. This maneuver is often helpful and essential when placing the prosthesis in awake patients to facilitate the engagement of the posterior margin of the perforation. The nasal mucosa is appropriately decongested and topically anesthetized, and a 0° endoscope can be used to assist in placing large buttons. The prosthesis is introduced through patients' right nostril; the posterior phalanges are seated into the posterior margin; the left anterior flange is moved into the left side of the nose with a forceps, suction tip, or elevator. The sutures are then cut and removed, and the rigid endoscope is used to ensure the superior flanges are medial to the middle turbinates (**Fig. 3**). If the prosthetic design

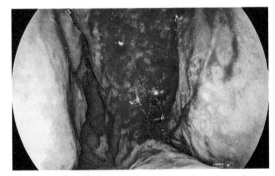

Fig. 2. The operative endoscopic examination of the perforation, after crust removal, of the patient whose CT is shown in **Fig. 1**. This patient has concurrent left inferior turbinate hypertrophy narrowing the airway.

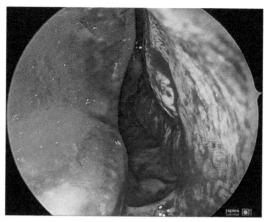

Fig. 3. Showing the same patient as in **Figs. 1** and **2** after placement of the custom button and submucosal reduction of the left inferior turbinate. Note the closely conforming fit of the wide posterior, superior margin, and the extension of the button down over the left maxillary crest.

created flanges that are too long at the time of placement, the prosthesis can be removed, trimmed, and replaced in the same fashion.

Patient Satisfaction

The authors recently published their prosthesis retention rates from 3 different patient populations, each using a different sizing methodology.[10] The first group included the time period up to 1982, at the beginning of CT sizing, and primarily used other methods, such as dye on paper to size the defects.[8] The second group extended from 1982 up to 2003 with prostheses sized using 2D reconstruction.[1] The third is the most recent group, which used 3D printed templates, starting in 2007.[10] In all 3 of the series, patients reported comparable improvements in symptoms; however, each series had a different retention rate. It was also noted that 7 patients kept their 3D-sized prosthesis after a failed prosthetic closure using a previous sizing method.[10]

For the 3D-sized patients, the average greatest diameter of the perforation was 2.4 cm and the average area of the defect was 3.1 cm^2. Nineteen of the 21 (90%) patients retained their prostheses at 7 to 51 months of follow-up.[10] In the series whereby the perforations were sized by a paper template, the retention rate for closure was 73% (100 of 136).[8] For the series reported in 2003, all sized by CT in 2D, the retention rate was 77% (57 of 74).[1]

LIMITATIONS

The evolution in the design process for prosthetic closure of nasal septal perforations has resulted in a prosthesis with a more precise fit and optimal patient comfort. It successfully covers all of the perforation's tissue margins and minimizes symptoms, particularly those of crusting and bleeding, but can still feel obstructive in some patients. Consideration for inferior turbinate reduction may be made in patients with obstruction despite good closure.

As 3D printers become more affordable, the option of using the technology for designing custom buttons will become more widespread. A good interdisciplinary relationship between the otolaryngology, radiology, and prosthetic departments is crucial for the success of this exacting process. As 3D printing advances, many of the intermediate steps will likely be eliminated and we may have the ability to directly print medical-grade prostheses, tissue scaffolds,[11] or even 3D-printed stem cell generating tissue[12–14] that will be placed to replete the missing septal tissue in situ.[15]

SUMMARY

Successful closure of nasal septal perforations, surgical or prosthetic, can provide significant improvement in the disease-specific symptoms. Using 3D printing technology to precisely size a nasal septal perforation allows for a more optimal prosthesis fit. Preliminary data reveal a 90% retention rate suggesting that these custom buttons are more comfortable, especially in patients with large and irregular perforations.

REFERENCES

1. Price DL, Sherris DA, Kern EB. Computed tomography for constructing custom nasal septal buttons. Arch Otolaryngol 2003;129:1236–9.
2. Meyer R. Neuerungen in der Nasenplastik. Practica Otolaryngol 1951;13:373–6.
3. Kim SW, Rhee CS. Nasal septal perforation repair: predictive factors and systematic review of the literature. Curr Opin Otolaryngol Head Neck Surg 2012;20: 58–65.
4. Moon IJ, Kim SW, Han DH, et al. Predictive factors for the outcome of nasal septal perforation repair. Auris Nasus Larynx 2011;38:52–7.
5. Kern EB, Facer GW, McDonald TJ, et al. Closure of nasal septal perforations with a Silastic button. ORL Digest 1977;39:9–17.
6. Facer GW, Kern EB. Nasal septal perforations: use of Silastic button in 108 patients. Rhinology 1979;17:115–20.
7. Facer GW, Kern EB. Nonsurgical closure of nasal septal perforations. Arch Otolaryngol 1979;105:6–8.
8. Pallanch JF, Facer GW, Kern EB, et al. Prosthetic closure of nasal septal perforations. Otolaryngol Head Neck Surg 1982;90:448–52.
9. Arbour P. "How I do it"–head and neck: a targeted problem and its solution. Practical suggestion in cases of septal perforation: an easy way to insert the Kern's septal obturator. Laryngoscope 1979;89:1170–1.
10. Onerci Altunay Z, Bly JA, Edwards PK, et al. Three-dimensional printing of large nasal septal perforations for optimal prosthetic closure. Am J Rhinol Allergy 2016; 30:287–93.
11. Maciulaitis J, Deveikyte M, Rekstyte S, et al. Preclinical study of SZ2080 material 3D microstructured scaffolds for cartilage tissue engineering made by femtosecond direct laser writing lithography. Biofabrication 2015;7:015015.
12. Younesi M, Islam A, Kishore V, et al. Fabrication of compositionally and topographically complex robust tissue forms by 3D-electrochemical compaction of collagen. Biofabrication 2015;7:035001.
13. Ouyang L, Yao R, Chen X, et al. 3D printing of HEK 293FT cell-laden hydrogel into macroporous constructs with high cell viability and normal biological functions. Biofabrication 2015;7:015010.
14. Zhao Y, Li Y, Mao S, et al. The influence of printing parameters on cell survival rate and printability in microextrusion-based 3D cell printing technology. Biofabrication 2015;7:045002.
15. Sharma A, Janus JR, Hamilton GS. Regenerative medicine and nasal surgery. Mayo Clin Proc 2015;90:148–58.

Advances in Microdebrider Technology

Improving Functionality and Expanding Utility

Dennis Tang, MD[a], Brian C. Lobo, MD[a], Brian D'Anza, MD[b],
Troy D. Woodard, MD[a], Raj Sindwani, MD, FACS[a],*

KEYWORDS

- Microdebrider • Powered instrumentation • Endoscopic • Sinus surgery
- Skull base surgery • Polyps • Drill

KEY POINTS

- Microdebriders are an essential tool in modern endoscopic sinus surgery.
- Angled blades allow for easier access to portions of the maxillary and frontal sinuses.
- There have been recent adaptations in microdebrider design for application in endoscopic skull base surgery and in-office use.
- Because of the high suction and speed of powered instrumentation, safe techniques must be used to avoid injury to the skull base, orbit and adjacent structures.

UPDATES ON MICRODEBRIDER TECHNOLOGY

Microdebrider technology has revolutionized the way endoscopic sinus surgery (ESS) is performed. The advantages of an instrument that can simultaneously suction and remove tissue include decreased operative time, improved precision and visualization, and expedited removal of diseased tissue.

The surgical predecessor to the microdebrider dates back to the mid 1960s, when Dr Jack Urban of the House Ear Institute envisioned a rotary vacuum dissector that could be used for controlled removal of tissue in a cramped surgical field. After securing a patent in 1969, it was used initially by Dr William House for resection of acoustic neuromas through the 1970s, ultimately gaining popularity with orthopedic surgeons for arthroscopic procedures in the 1980s.[1] It was not until the mid-1990s that the microdebrider made its way to otolaryngology, when Setliff and Parsons[2]

[a] Section of Rhinology and Skull Base Surgery, Minimally Invasive Cranial Base & Pituitary Surgery Program, Head and Neck Institute, Burkhardt Brain Tumor and Neuro-Oncology Center, Cleveland Clinic Foundation, 9500 Euclid Avenue #A-71, Cleveland, OH 44195, USA; [b] Section of Rhinology and Skull Base Surgery, Department of Otolaryngology, University Hospitals–Case Western Reserve University, 11100 Euclid Avenue, Cleveland, OH 44106, USA
* Corresponding author.
E-mail address: sindwar@ccf.org

Otolaryngol Clin N Am 50 (2017) 589–598
http://dx.doi.org/10.1016/j.otc.2017.01.009
0030-6665/17/© 2017 Elsevier Inc. All rights reserved.

described using the "Hummer," a microdebrider then produced by Stryker, for use in ESS.

BASIC FUNCTION

Since Setliff's description in 1994, microdebrider technology has continued to evolve and has become indispensable in the rhinologist's surgical armamentarium. The basic design of the microdebrider consists of a reuseable hand piece connected to a suction source, an interchangeable blade, a power unit, and a control foot switch. The interchangeable blade connects to the hand piece and is usually disposable. It typically consists of 2 hollow concentric shafts: a fixed outer shaft with a port for tissue to enter, and a rotating (or oscillating) inner shaft designed with a cutting surface. When the ports on the inner and outer shafts align, soft tissue is drawn into the inner lumen via suction, and as the inner blade rotates or oscillates, the trapped tissue within the port is sheared off and immediately suctioned from the field through the inner lumen of the blade and ultimately the hand piece. These removed pieces of tissue can be captured in a downstream trap for subsequent histopathologic analysis. Irrigation is typically integrated into the device, applied by a separate set of tubing, and pumped into the blade to facilitate movement of debrided tissue. The irrigation helps to prevent clogging of the device by the aspirated tissue and debris.

Although multiple modes have been developed for the microdebrider, the blades ultimately rotate or oscillate. Oscillation is typically used for soft tissue resection as the slower speed operation (up to 5000 revolutions per minute, rpm) allows for more soft tissue to be drawn into the inner lumen before the inner blade cuts the tissue. The slower the oscillation speed, the longer the suction phase of the aperture's cycle, and the more aggressively the device functions. Rotation can also be used for soft tissue removal, but typically the rotational mode is now preferred for use with endoscopic burr attachments. Contemporary systems offer multi-instrument consoles, which permit several powered instruments (drills, shavers, and so forth) to be plugged into and run off of the same hardware platform. "Smart" consoles actually will recognize the type of blade that is inserted into the connected hand piece and even recall surgeon preferences for settings.

SPECIALTY BLADES

Improvement in blade design has allowed for efficient tissue removal, augmented access to sinuses, expeditious bone removal, and the ability to use the microdebrider to address turbinate hypertrophy and even septal spurs.

Blade Opening

Various blade configurations of the microdebrider have emerged for specific applications. Initially, microdebrider blades were designed with a rectangular opening; however this shape has evolved over time to include clover shaped openings as the rectangular ones were found to clog easily. The cloverleaf design better morselizes tissue into smaller pieces. Blade diameter ranges from 2 mm to 4 mm, with larger blades resulting in less clogging and more efficient debridement. However, larger blades limit maneuverability in restricted cavities, and careful consideration must be taken when selecting the blade for each application. The traditional cutting surface is straight-edged, allowing for precise and careful dissection with minimal trauma to adjacent tissue. Development of a serrated edge allowed for better gripping of soft tissue and more aggressive debridement.

The newest straight blade from Medtronic (Jacksonville, FL, USA) is the Quadcut design with a cloverleaf-shaped opening and a slightly larger outer diameter

(4.3 mm) in comparison to the older Tricut blade (4.0 mm) (**Fig. 1**). Studies using analogs to nasal polyps and allergic fungal sinusitis showed reduced clog frequency and decreased operative time when using the Quadcut blade compared with the Tricut blade.[3] The newest Olympus (Center Valley, PA, USA) Diego Elite device allows for effective and rapid declogging by using an in-line pneumatic squeeze bulb feature (**Fig. 2**).

Angled Blades

Endoscopic access to the maxillary sinus with a straight cannula microdebrider is restricted to the antrum and immediate posterior wall. Full access to the sinus mucosa is necessary for entities such as inverted papilloma or malignant lesions. Access to the maxilla in these situations may require a large antrostomy or conversion to an open technique. The recent development of specific angled blades (Medtronic RAD line; **Fig. 3**) has improved access to a greater proportion of the maxillary sinus. These angles include 12, 40, 60, 90, and 120 for the Medtronic RAD line and 15, 40, 60, 75, and 90 for the Olympus Diego device. Cadaver studies have shown access to 81% of the maxillary mucosa surface area through a 1-cm × 1-cm antrostomy when using angled blades.[4] The angles used for this study included 15, 40, 70, and 120. However, accessing most of the sinus required the use of multiple different angled blades, potentially increasing the cost of the procedure. These angled blades allow reliable entry into the frontal recess, permitting complete access to all the paranasal sinuses with a single tool. It should be noted that access to the anterior maxillary sinus and the far lateral reaches of the frontal sinus are still very challenging even with appropriate instrumentation.

Turbinectomy and Septoplasty Blades

Blades designed for specific submucosal resection of the septum or septal spurs as well as inferior turbinates allow for resection of specific portions of bony and cartilaginous structures with minimal injury to the mucosa. These blades are small in diameter, measuring 2.0 or 2.9 mm, and some offer a beveled guard on the back of the blade to aid in dissection and protect the turbinate mucosa. In some microdebriders, the instrument tip is hooded and sharp enough to create the initial stab incision, reducing the need to switch between instruments.

NAVIGATION

Image guidance has been a major boon for endoscopic sinus surgeons, especially in the setting of revision surgery or advanced skull base surgery. The first interactive image guidance systems were developed in the 1980s but were difficult to configure and

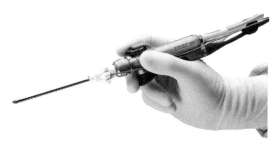

Fig. 1. Image of Medtronic M5 with Quad blade. (*Reprinted* with the permission of Medtronic, Inc. © 2016.)

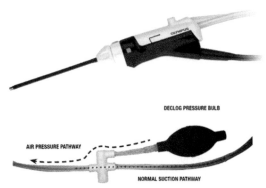

Fig. 2. Olympus Diego Elite device with rapid declogging bulb. (*Courtesy of* Olympus, Center Valley, PA; with permission.)

required head fixation using a frame. The advent of high-resolution computed tomography combined with the development of electromagnetic (EM) and optical localization transformed the navigation technology by making it widely accessible and easily usable by surgical teams. Current interactive computer imaging systems allow for faster registration, greater accuracy, and less morbidity, with described navigation accuracy of 2 mm or less.[5] This finding is independent of proprietary fiducial markers.

Interactive image guidance affords the ability to correlate surgical anatomy with 3-dimensional radiologic findings in real time. Image guidance significantly decreases the dependence on radiographic images placed on the wall or on light boxes and allows the surgeon to focus on the patient with all information at the ready.

Microdebrider technology has advanced with the newest systems integrating optical or EM technologies. These blades include those compatible with Medtronic M4 and M5 series microdebriders as well as those for the Olympus Diego (PK and Elite) devices. It should be noted that for the Medtronic devices, this is incorporated into the blade itself and makes easy use of their Fusion system as a "plug and play" attachment. The Olympus devices marry with an optical-based navigation platform via a reflector array on a post that screws directly onto the back of the microdebrider

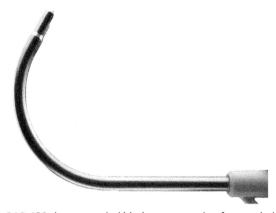

Fig. 3. Medtronic RAD 120-degree angled blade, an example of an angled blade. (*Reprinted with the permission of Medtronic, Inc. © 2016.*)

hand piece (**Fig. 4**) and integrates with the BrainLab (Feldkirche, Germany) navigation system. Navigation allows tip localization in 3 dimensions and can predict the trajectory of the instrument. Use of an image-guided microdebrider is certainly helpful for orientation during revision procedures, frontal dissection, tumor removal, and cases with significant anatomic variance.

Recent surveys show an increasing trend of image guidance availability and use in otolaryngology practices.[6] Objective evidence that image-guidance systems provide additional safety to ESS is lacking in contemporary studies, possibly due to the overall decrease in complication rates as the field has matured and training and anatomic understanding have improved. It is critical to remember that image guidance systems are not perfect and nothing will substitute for thorough knowledge of anatomy. If there is any discord between anatomic and image guidance findings, care should be taken to ensure reliability as fiducial markers may have shifted during surgery.

DRILL BURR ATTACHMENTS

Initial microdebriders were limited by low revolution speeds, with the "Hummer" device limited to 1600 rpm. Although this was sufficient for soft tissue removal, expanded ESS techniques have advanced such that bone removal during procedures is common. In this vein, rotational speed has increased with each iteration of microdebrider technology, with the Olympus device the industry leader at 15,000 rpm for years. The most recent generation of Medtronic microdebriders, however, allow for speeds of up to 30,000 rpm. With these higher speeds, endoscopic burrs are now more effective in removing thicker bone and have found applications in Draf III procedures, septoplasty, endoscopic dacryocystorhinostomy, and fibro-osseous tumor removal. A major advantage of the high speeds now available is the associated cost and time savings, as one no longer requires a separate endoscopic drill or multiple blades/burrs to be used with each case.

Available burr heads include cutting burrs, diamond burrs, and shielded burrs available in both straight and curved designs (**Fig. 5**). These burrs are capable of precise removal of bone and are self-irrigating.

ENERGY-EQUIPPED BLADES

Microdebriders allow multitasking. Their greatest utility comes from the fact that they provide continuous suctioning of blood from the surgical field while allowing expeditious tissue removal. The dual functionality microdebriders was heralded as a major advance in ESS performed for polyp or tumor removal, which can be quite bloody. Interestingly, although they provide better visualization of the field for the operator, conventional microdebriders do nothing to actually stop the bleeding. A recent improvement in microdebrider functionality has been the incorporation of energy into the tips of the

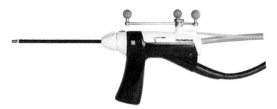

Fig. 4. Image of Olympus Diego Elite device. (*Courtesy* of Olympus, Center Valley, PA; with permission.)

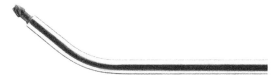

Fig. 5. Example of Medtronic cutting burr attachment for drilling. (*Reprinted* with the permission of Medtronic, Inc. © 2016.)

blades for the purpose of providing hemostasis during a procedure. The Olympus platform was the first to incorporate the delivery of bipolar or monopolar energy to the end of the microdebrider blade (**Fig. 6**). The current blade design includes inner and outer electrodes surrounded by an insulation layer so that the energy is delivered around the aperture of the blade providing accurate delivery of cautery with limited thermal spread (see **Fig. 6**). However, the small size of the bipolar cautery zone makes it difficult to control brisk bleeding, and the monopolar energy source is thought to be more effective. In the clinical setting of exposed neurovital structures (brain, orbit, and so forth), however, monopolar cautery is relatively contraindicated, and the use of bipolar energy is advised. A prospective, controlled study of 80 patients undergoing surgery for chronic rhinosinusitis with polyps showed that the use of the PK Diego system equipped with bipolar energy significantly reduced blood loss and operative time compared with a conventional microdebrider.[7] The new generation of Diego devices has some integrated distal suction that continuously clears blood while administering bipolar cautery. The Diego Elite system is presently the only microdebrider that incorporates electrocautery into its blades. Emerging applications for this type of technology include ESS, turbinate reduction, adenoidectomy, and even skull base surgery.

SKULL BASE APPLICATIONS

Endoscopic treatment of skull base tumors is an exciting area of development in rhinology. Development of microdebrider devices designed specifically for resection of intracranial masses through the narrow endonasal corridor is a recent development. The NICO Myriad (NICO Corp., Indianapolis, IN, USA) is a novel device specifically created for this application (**Fig. 7**). This shaving device has a high-speed

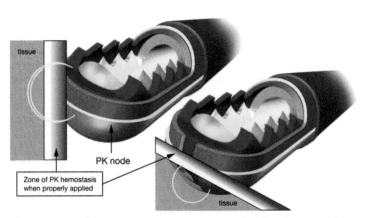

Fig. 6. Implementation of Olympus Diego Elite cauterization showing area of heat conduction. (*Courtesy of* Olympus, Center Valley, PA; with permission.)

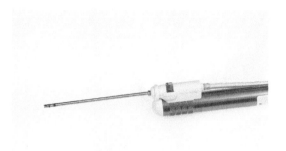

Fig. 7. NICO Myriad skull base tumor debridement device. (*Courtesy of* NICO Corporation, Indianapolis, IN; with permission.)

reciprocating inner cannula positioned inside a stationary outer cannula with an electronically controlled variable suction. There is an integrated blunt dissector end that is located distal to the aspiration aperture. The greatest advantage of this device is the ability to precisely control suction strength by graded depression of the foot pedal or a knob on the console. It is also malleable, although to a limited extent, and comes in several lengths and diameters. Importantly, suction can be immediately stopped by releasing actuation of the foot pedal to avoid cutting tissue that may have been inadvertently suctioned into the aperture. This device has been shown in case series to be effective in removal of fibrous pituitary adenomas, craniopharyngiomas, and loculated hydrocephalus.[8] The ability to resect, suction, and bluntly dissect in one integrated tool makes tissue resection more efficient compared with existing endoscopic instrumentation, avoiding the need to switch between tools. There also appears to be a safety advantage when operating in a confined space flanked by exposed neurovital structures as is routinely encountered during intracranial surgery. Disadvantages of the device include lack of hemostatic capability, difficulty removing extremely fibrous tumors, and significant associated cost. Further development of modified microdebrider technologies for use during endoscopic intracranial surgery is a trend that is sure to continue.

IN-OFFICE PROCEDURES

Until recently, most sinus surgery was performed in the operating room setting under general anesthesia. With the increased focus on health care spending and costs, a growing trend of procedures is now being seen moving from the higher cost operating room environment to the lower cost in-office setting. In-office procedures benefits to the patient (lower risk, as it avoids general anesthesia, minimal recovery time), the surgeon (easier to schedule, less involved), and the entire health system (significant cost savings), so long as similar goals of disease management and patient outcomes can be accomplished.

Dovetailing on the proliferation of in-office balloon procedures, some microdebrider technologies are now catering specifically to soft tissue/polyp removal for the in-office setting. In 2014, a solely vacuum-powered disposable microdebrider called the PolypVac (Laurimed, Redwood City, CA, USA) was approved by the US Food and Drug Administration for in-office polypectomy. This device is a one-time use, disposable unit with a reciprocating (guillotine) motion similar to the NICO Myriad device (**Fig. 8**). Key advantages of this device over the traditional electric-powered

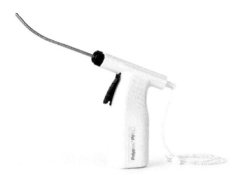

Fig. 8. Polpvac vacuum-based in-office polypectomy device. (*Courtesy of* Laurimed, Redwood City, CA; with permission.)

microdebrider for the clinic setting are its quick setup, cost, and simplicity. The device is entirely powered via a suction line, and there is an irrigation line connected to a syringe filled with sterile water or saline to prevent clogging with no need for a console, foot pedal, or separate mounting pole. In addition, the tip is malleable, allowing the microdebrider to be bent at different angles needed to maximize access to different areas or sinuses all with one device. Notable disadvantages include its lack of power or speed compared with the electric devices (making it slower and less robust), which results in a decreased ability to resect more fibrous polyps and tissue, and its inability to take down bone (even small partitions encountered in the ethmoid, for example). Thus, the application of the vacuum-powered microdebrider is best directed toward patients with recurrent nasal polyposis who have previously undergone ESS or the patient with polyps restricted to the nasal cavity. A recent retrospective case series showed most patients tolerated in-office polypectomy well, with 87% of the procedures considered a success.[9] Forty-three percent of patients described improvement in nasal obstruction. The primary failure was secondary to fibrous polyps in 10% of cases.

LIMITATIONS

Similar to any other device, there are limitations to the use of microdebriders that must be recognized for safe and proper use. The microdebriders are powered, suction-equipped devices that are very efficient at removing tissue. It is imperative that the surgeon recognize that there is reduced tactile feedback with the microdebrider in comparison to conventional hand-held instrumentation. This decrease in tactile feedback is most pronounced with removing soft tissue compared with bony structures. Care must be taken to ensure tissue is not removed inappropriately.

The use of microdebriders in the paranasal sinuses in close proximity to the orbit and skull base has raised concern for safety of these tools in ESS. Chou and colleagues[10] performed a study in 2016 addressing complications from ESS. Among 997 patients who underwent ESS with 487 patients using microdebrider and 510 patients with traditional instrumentation, there were no differences in complications rates. Overall complication rates are around 7.8%, including postoperative bleeding, breach of lamina papyracea, orbital cellulitis, and high-volume blood loss. Major complication rates remain low at 0.5%, consisting of cerebrospinal fluid leak, retrobulbar hematoma, and damage to medial rectus muscle. There is a recent sobering case report describing a patient who suffered complete enucleation of the orbit during

ESS.[11] It is critical to remember that the rate of tissue removal with the microdebrider is accelerated in comparison to conventional instrumentation, which can lead to faster progression of complications. Failure to rapidly recognize violation of anatomic boundaries can lead to devastating complications.

There is also an associated cost with the use of microdebriders, albeit variable. Most blades are designed to be single-use, disposable devices. Additional adjunct devices, including irrigation and suction, must also be added separately. Despite the added cost of a powered instrument, there is significant operative time reduction with the microdebrider. A randomized controlled trial in the Netherlands used ESS for chronic rhinosinusitis with nasal polyposis with bilateral uncinectomy, anterior and posterior ethmoidectomy, and Draf IIa or sphenoidectomy, if necessary, using conventional instrumentation on one side and microdebrider on the other side.[12] This study showed a significant decrease in operative time from 41 minutes with the traditional instrumentation in comparison to 30 minutes with the microdebrider. There was no difference in blood loss, pain, or recovery time. The decrease in operative time makes the microdebrider a cost-effective tool in appropriate applications.

SUMMARY

Microdebriders have dramatically advanced the field of ESS. Recent advances have expanded the application of microdebriders to improve access to all sinuses, and increase rotational speed for drilling, addition of energy for hemostasis capability, removal of skull base masses, and in-office polypectomy. As the functionality and utility of microdebriders expand, it becomes increasingly important to understand proper use and limitations of these devices to maintain safety and avoid complications.

REFERENCES

1. Krouse HJ, Parker CM, Purcell R, et al. Powered functional endoscopic sinus surgery. AORN J 1997;66(3):405–14.
2. Setliff RC, Parsons DS. The "Hummer": new instrumentation for functional endoscopic sinus surgery. Am J Rhinology 1994;8(6):275–8.
3. Boone JL, Feldt BA, McmAins KC, et al. Improved function of prototype 4.3-mm Medtronic Quadcut microdebrider blade over standard 4.0-mm Medtronic Tricut microdebrider blade. Int Forum Allergy Rhinol 2011;1(3):198–200.
4. Beswick DM, Rodriguez KD, Olds CE, et al. Quantification of maxillary sinus accessibility via a middle meatal antrostomy. Am J Rhinol Allergy 2015;29(5): 394–6.
5. Labadie RF, Davis BM, Fitzpatrick JM. Image-guided surgery: what is the accuracy? Curr Opin Otolaryngol Head Neck Surg 2005;13(1):27–31.
6. Justice JM, Orlandi RR. An update on attitudes of image-guided surgery. Int Forum Allergy Rhinol 2012;2(2):155–9.
7. Kumar N, Sindwani R. Bipolar microdebrider may reduce intraoperative blood loss and operative time during nasal polyp surgery. Ear Nose Throat J 2012; 91(8):336–44.
8. Dloughy BJ, Dahdaleh NS, Greenlee JDW. Emerging technology in intracranial neuroendoscopy: application of the NICO Myriad. Neurosurg Focus 2011; 30(4):1–9.
9. Gan EC, Habib AR, Hathorn I, et al. The efficacy and safety of an office-based polypectomy with a vacuum-powered microdebrider. Int Forum Allergy Rhinol 2013;3:890–5.

10. Chou TW, Chen PS, Lin HC, et al. Multiple analyses of factors related to complications in endoscopic sinus surgery. J Chin Med Assoc 2016;79:88–92.
11. Chang JR, Grant MP, Merbs SL. Enucleation as endoscopic sinus surgery complication. JAMA Ophthalmol 2015;133(7):850–2.
12. Cornet ME, Reinartz SM, Georgalas C, et al. The microdebrider, a step forward or an expensive gadget? Rhinology 2012;50:191–8.

Emerging Roles of Coblation in Rhinology and Skull Base Surgery

 CrossMark

Garret W. Choby, MD, Peter H. Hwang, MD*

KEYWORDS

- Coblation • Bipolar radiofrequency • Microdebrider • Endoscopic sinus surgery
- Skull base surgery • Blood loss • Complications • Outcomes

KEY POINTS

- Coblation is a type of bipolar radiofrequency ablation that works at relatively low temperatures by disrupting molecular bonds and allowing tissues to dissolve.
- Coblation may be associated with less postoperative pain following submucosal inferior turbinate reduction than other alternative techniques. Its duration of effect may be shorter than alternative surgical options.
- Additional applications in sinonasal and skull base surgery are actively being investigated (nasal polyposis, encephaloceles, juvenile nasal angiofibromas, skull base malignancies). Some studies have demonstrated a reduction in blood loss and improved endoscopic visualization.
- The cost of Coblation is often higher than that of traditional instruments. The benefits and costs of this technology must be carefully balanced.
- Longer-term outcomes studies for the various indications for Coblation are necessary to guide surgical decision making regarding Coblation therapies.

INTRODUCTION

Radiofrequency (RF) tissue ablation has been used safely and effectively for years in several surgical fields, including neurosurgery, urology, and gynecology. More recently, this technology has been applied to otolaryngologic procedures.[1] Within otolaryngology, this technique has been used most commonly for tonsil and adenoid surgery. Additional roles within the sinonasal cavity, however, are actively being investigated.

Disclosure Statement: The authors have no commercial interest or conflicts of interest to report.
Division of Rhinology and Endoscopic Skull Base Surgery, Department of Otolaryngology–Head and Neck Surgery, Stanford University, 801 Welch Road, MC 5739, Stanford, CA 94305, USA
* Corresponding author.
E-mail address: hwangph@stanford.edu

Otolaryngol Clin N Am 50 (2017) 599–606
http://dx.doi.org/10.1016/j.otc.2017.01.010
0030-6665/17/© 2017 Elsevier Inc. All rights reserved.

Two distinct types of RF ablation exist, unipolar and bipolar. Most applications described here use bipolar RF technology. Coblation (Arthrocare ENT, Sunnyvale, CA; USA) is a specific type of bipolar RF ablation that works by creating a low-temperature sodium chloride RF plasma field between bipolar electrodes. This energy disrupts molecular bonds, allowing tissues to dissolve. This controlled ablation, or "Coblation," allows ablation of tissue to occur at relatively low temperatures (typically 60–70°C), which is thought to limit thermal damage to surrounding tissues with a depth of penetration of 2 to 4 mm.[2,3] On the other hand, unipolar RF devices deliver energy to the tip of the device, which is then dispersed into the surrounding tissue. Depth of penetration of unipolar RF is greater than bipolar RF and can be up to 20 mm.[3–5] Furthermore, unipolar RF requires that a grounding electrode be placed on the patient.

Coblation has been adapted for use within the sinonasal cavity, including treatment of adenoids, inferior turbinates, nasal polyps, encephaloceles, and skull base tumors. Although still under investigation, potential benefits of Coblation include reduced blood loss, improved visualization, and reduced thermal injury to surrounding tissue. The main limitations are cost, potential adverse effects on functional epithelium, and relative paucity of long-term outcomes.

COBLATION FOR INFERIOR TURBINATE SURGERY

Inferior turbinate (IT) hypertrophy is a leading cause of nasal airway obstruction and a frequent site of targeted surgical interventions. IT hypertrophy is associated with allergic rhinitis, vasomotor rhinitis, and nasal septum deviation (compensatory).[5] A variety of topical medications, including corticosteroid nasal sprays, may help to alleviate symptoms, but surgery is often indicated in refractory cases. Numerous techniques have been described, including turbinectomy, laser-assisted turbinoplasty, monopolar and bipolar cautery, and submucosal IT reduction. Submucosal reduction is often preferred because it is mucosal sparing and thus more likely to preserve the physiologic functions of the turbinate, including humidification and warming of inspired air. Overresection of the inferior turbinates may predispose the patient to dryness, crusting, atrophic rhinitis, or paradoxic nasal obstruction (empty nose syndrome).[5–7] Common methods used for submucosal IT reduction include microdebrider resection, monopolar RF ablation, and Coblation.

Coblation is thought to achieve volumetric reduction of the submucosal IT tissue via 2 mechanisms: tissue ablation as an immediate effect of applying RF energy and postoperative tissue contraction as a delayed effect of wound healing. Histologic changes after Coblation treatment of the IT tissue include decreased submucosal glands and decreased venous sinusoids. However, there may also be epithelial disruption and shedding.[8]

Clinical outcomes of Coblation submucosal IT reduction have been studied in several articles. Hegazy and colleagues[9] examined the outcomes of patients treated with endoscopic-assisted submucosal IT reduction with Coblation versus microdebrider in a prospective randomized trial. Forty patients were treated in the Coblation group (Coblator II System; Arthrocare), and 30 patients were treated in the microdebrider group (Medtronic, Jacksonville, FL, USA). Patients in the microdebrider group had increased pain postoperatively at 48 hours compared with the Coblation group ($P<.001$). No other outcome measures (postoperative adhesions, duration of surgery, or symptom improvement) reached statistical significance. Both groups maintained IT size reduction and symptom reduction at 6 months postoperatively ($P<.001$). However, a longer-term, randomized comparison of Coblation versus microdebrider IT reduction examined both subjective and objective outcomes. Subjective measurements included nasal obstruction, sneezing rhinorrhea, and snoring, while objective measures included nasal resistance and saccharin transit time. There were comparable improvements in both groups over the first year after treatment. However, there was evidence of regression of clinical benefit in the Coblation group between 1 to 3 years, whereas the microdebrider group reported sustained improvement for the 3 years of follow-up.[10]

The observation that the therapeutic effects of Coblation may peak at the first year was also echoed in a study by Passali and colleagues,[11] who examined outcomes of submucosal IT reduction using Coblation versus unipolar RF ablation. Coblation was carried out in 25 patients and unipolar RF ablation in 15 patients; all patients were followed for 3 years postoperatively. Both groups showed improvement after 1 year in regards to anterior rhinomanometry, acoustic rhinometry, and symptoms based on visual analogue scale. There were no significant differences between the 2 groups. It was noted, however, that both techniques showed diminishing benefit with regards to nasal resistance and nasal volume in the long term. About 50% of patients in both groups experienced a worsening in their nasal resistance and volume at 3-year follow-up compared with the 1-year follow-up, with no differences between the Coblation and unipolar RF groups. Scores at 3 years were still better than preoperative scores, however.

Another study examined postoperative outcomes of patients undergoing submucosal IT reduction using Coblation versus intramural bipolar cautery under local anesthesia. Forty-one patients were included in the study. All patients had submucosal Coblation performed on one IT and intramural bipolar cautery on the contralateral IT. Patients were followed for 6 weeks postoperatively. Both techniques had similar subjective and objective outcomes in nasal obstruction as measured by acoustic rhinometry and subjective visual analogue scales. Coblation was significantly less painful than intramural bipolar cautery during the procedure ($P = .03$) and during the immediate postoperative period ($P = .02$). There was also less crusting in the Coblation side at 3 weeks postoperatively ($P = .009$).[12] They concluded that both techniques result in similar overall outcomes, although the Coblation may result in less pain and less crusting in the early postoperative period. However, the study was limited by a very short follow-up period.

Regarding IT procedures in the pediatric population, a recent article examined practice patterns of member of the American Society of Pediatric Otolaryngologists pertaining to IT surgery. In this group of respondents, Coblation was the most common technique used for submucosal IT reduction (51% of respondents).[13] This use of Coblation differs significantly from a similar survey to the American Society of Plastic Surgeons examining trends in treatment of ITs during rhinoplasty. The largest portion of the respondents performed simple outfracture (49.1%), whereas a small minority used submucosal Coblation (5.6%) or submucosal microdebrider reduction (2.2%).[14] A similar survey has not been published among rhinologists.

Submucosal IT reduction with Coblation is increasing in popularity and may decrease postoperative discomfort and crusting compared with alternative techniques. The duration of effect appears to peak within the first year, and thus, patients should be counseled accordingly to create appropriate expectations regarding outcome. As most studies examining Coblation treatment of IT hypertrophy are limited in size and power, higher-level evidence is needed before definitive recommendations can be made.

COBLATION IN ENDOSCOPIC SINUS SURGERY

Eloy and colleagues[15] examined the use of Coblation-assisted endoscopic sinus surgery (ESS) for nasal polyposis. Twenty-one patients underwent endoscopic debulking of their polyps with Coblation followed by the standard indicated ESS with microdebrider, whereas 16 patients underwent endoscopic polyp debulking with a standard microdebrider (Diego-powered microdebrider; Olympus ENT, Bartlett, TN, USA) followed by the indicated ESS. All preoperative demographic and disease-specific data were similar. There were no significant outcome differences (estimated blood loss [EBL], EBL/min, operative time) between the Coblation and microdebrider groups in cases of primary polypectomy. However, in cases of revision polypectomy, the Coblator group had a significant reduction in EBL (307.1 mL vs 227.8 mL; $P = .0001$) and EBL/min of surgical time when compared with the microdebrider group (2.8 mL/min vs 4.8 mL/min; $P = .001$). Postoperative outcomes, such as crusting, pain, and ease of in-office debridements, were not studied.

Although the aforementioned study evaluated Coblation-assisted debulking of polyps as a prelude to ESS, there are a limited number of studies that have examined the use of Coblation for actual tissue dissection during ESS. When considering applying any type of energy to assist in surgical dissection of the sinuses, it is important to understand the depth of penetration of the applied energy as well as any effects the applied energy may have on healing epithelium. This understanding is particularly important in the sinuses, where preservation of functional mucosa is paramount and excessive depth of energy penetration may adversely affect critical adjacent structures, such as the orbit and brain. The effects of Coblation on nasal respiratory mucosa during simulated ESS have been investigated in rabbit and sheep models.[16,17] The Coblator was used to perform a simulated ESS on the animal (application of the Coblator wand to the IT as well as the lateral nasal wall and lamina papyracea for various durations of time). Microscopic examination of the tissue was undertaken after necropsy. Sheep were sacrificed immediately postoperatively or at 14 days postoperatively. Rabbits were sacrificed at postoperative day 3, 7, 14, and 29 (2 rabbits at each assigned day). In the rabbit model, the site of Coblation showed thermal damage to the epithelium and underlying seromucinous glands. Complete re-epithelialization occurred by postoperative day 29, but the seromucinous glands were replaced by fibrosis.[17] In the sheep model, similar results were found. The zone of thermal injury was no larger than the size of the Coblation wand with loss of epithelium and underlying seromucinous glands. The epithelium recovered with squamous metaplasia. Depth of thermal injury seemed to correspond to the type of submucosal tissue, not to the duration of the time in contact with the Coblator wand.[16] The authors thought that the Coblator created a limited zone of thermal injury.[16,17] These results suggest that Coblation can likely be used judiciously in the sinuses without adverse effects on the orbit or skull base. However, the fibrotic and metaplastic effects of Coblation suggest that it may be better suited to areas such as the turbinate, where fibrosis may be therapeutic, rather than the sinuses, where disruption of mucociliary clearance may affect functional outcomes. More studies are required to better delineate the tissue effects of Coblation.

COBLATION IN SKULL BASE SURGERY

The management of sinonasal and anterior skull base tumors has rapidly evolved over the past few decades. Large infiltrative tumors that would traditionally be resected with open approaches are increasingly being accessed from a minimally invasive endoscopic approach. In turn, technology has progressed with many advances allowing for improved visualization and access. One of the largest obstacles to safe and effective endoscopic skull base surgery is impaired visualization from tumor bleeding. Coblation has been applied in this setting to ablate tissue and reduce intraoperative blood loss, thus improving visualization.[18]

Kostrzewa and colleagues[18] examined the potential benefit of Coblation during endoscopic skull base tumor resection for decreasing blood loss. Because estimating blood loss during this type of surgery can be subjective and difficult to accurately record, they used an additional surrogate marker, the 11-point Wormald endoscopic surgical field grading scale. This scale has been shown to have higher interrater and intrarater reliability than previously described surgical field grading scales.[19] Twenty-three patients were included. In 13 patients, most of the tumor debulking was carried out with the microdebrider. In the remaining 10 patients, the Coblator was used. For tumors of similar size, Coblator-based tumor resection was associated with reduced EBL (350 mL vs 1000 mL; $P = .001$) and improvement in the Wormald surgical field grade score ($P = .001$). Although this was a small retrospective study, the investigators suggested that use of the Coblator may help to limit blood loss and improve visualization in select skull base tumors.[18]

Cannon and colleagues[20] described their experience with Coblation for juvenile nasopharyngeal angiofibroma (JNA) resection after preoperative embolization. JNAs are benign but local aggressive, highly vascular tumors that typically occur in adolescent men. Although not a comparative study, the investigators thought that the Coblator assisted with improved visualization and reduced EBL. These results are similar to a previously published case series of Coblation-assisted endoscopic resection of Fisch class I JNAs that examined 23 patients (12 patients with traditional endoscopic instruments; 11 patients with Coblation). They found that surgical time ($P<.001$) and EBL ($P<.001$) were reduced in the Coblation group.[21]

The use of the Coblator for endoscopic encephalocele reduction has also been studied. Nasal encephaloceles are herniations of meninges with brain tissue into the nasal cavity through a bony defect in the skull base. Bipolar electrocautery has traditionally been used to reduce these to decrease the risk of intracerebral bleeding. Smith and colleagues[22] described their experience with the Coblator for endoscopic reduction of encephaloceles in 19 patients compared with a historic cohort of 6 patients with encephaloceles reduced with bipolar electrocautery. Encephalocele size was comparable in both groups. They found that the encephalocele reduction time in the Coblator group was reduced compared with the bipolar group (15.8 minutes vs 46 minutes; $P = .0003$); there was no difference in the incidence of bleeding events.

The above limited studies show that there may be a role for Coblation in these cases to reduce EBL and thus improve endoscopic visualization. Before definitive conclusions can be drawn, however, additional study and investigation is warranted.

OTHER APPLICATIONS AND CONSIDERATIONS OF COBLATOR TECHNOLOGY

Coblation has been described as a tool to control epistaxis in patients with hereditary hemorrhagic telangiectasias (HHT). A variety of techniques have been used to address this difficult problem, including various lasers, bipolar cautery, microdebrider, septodermoplasty, and nasal closure (Young procedure).[23–26] Although KTP (potassium titanyl phosphate) laser ablation is arguably the gold standard, it is expensive and difficult to use in a bloody surgical field. Joshi and colleagues[4] described a case series of 5 patients with HHT who were treated with Coblation. Epistaxis control was achieved in 4 of 5 patients, with the fifth patient requiring packing, embolization, and subsequent Young procedure. Although no comparative trials have been undertaken between Coblation and other established methods of epistaxis control, Coblation may be considered as an additional tool in the arsenal of the rhinologist to treat this difficult disease.

Another more common rhinologic application of Coblation is adenoidectomy. There are many theoretic benefits including reduced pain and reduced blood loss. Although these potential benefits have not been well established in clinical trials, there is some mixed evidence that the Coblation method of adenoidectomy may reduce surgical time and blood loss. Kim and colleagues[27] conducted a prospective multicenter trial examining safety and outcomes of adenoidectomy with various surgical techniques. They concluded that Coblation-assisted adenoidectomy (Arthocare ENT, Stockholm, Sweden) resulted in shorter operative time ($P<.001$) and reduced EBL ($P<.001$) when compared with microdebrider-assisted adenoidectomy (Medtronic Xomed, Jacksonville, FL, USA) with and without cauterization. Thottam and colleagues[28] compared the cost and efficacy of 1280 cases of adenotonsillectomy using several surgical instruments, including monopolar cautery (Bovie monopolar cautery and suction bovie; Covidien, Dublin, Ireland), Coblation, and PlasmaBlade (Medtronic, Minneapolis, MN, USA). They noted a statistically significant reduced operative time in the monopolar cautery group compared with the Coblation group ($P = .001$) and PlasmaBlade group ($P = .03$). There was no difference in postoperative bleeding rates. At their institution, the average cost for the instrument was $30.04 for monopolar cautery, $246.95 for PlasmaBlade, and $244.32 for the Coblator.

In the current health care climate, the cost of various surgical instruments must be considered. Cost is a difficult factor to study, because monetary charges may vary among institutions. In addition, other downstream effects must be taken into account, such as operating room time and readmission rates. Although no specific studies primarily examine the cost of the Coblator for sinonasal procedures, a pediatric study examined cost differences for tonsillectomy when completed with electrocautery versus Coblation versus microdebrider. At their institution, the total nondisposable instrument costs for Coblation-assisted tonsillectomy were $1105.02 versus $730 for electrocautery versus $672.88 for microdebrider. The investigators argue that this difference in cost may potentially be justified based on reduced operating time and reduced postoperative symptoms.[29] As with all surgery, costs must be balanced with potential benefits of the technology.

SUMMARY

Coblation is a relatively new bipolar RF ablation tool that is gaining favor for some sinonasal surgical applications. Potential benefits may include reduced intraoperative bleeding, improved endoscopic visualization, and reduced pain. The main drawbacks are its relatively high cost and potential adverse effects on functional epithelium. At this juncture, most of the published evidence is promising, but low level. Further investigation is warranted to determine if the potential benefits outweigh the costs.

REFERENCES

1. Coste A, Yona L, Blumen M, et al. Radiofrequency is a safe and effective treatment of turbinate hypertrophy. Laryngoscope 2001;111(5):894–9.
2. Grobler A, Carney AS. Radiofrequency coblation tonsillectomy. Br J Hosp Med (Lond) 2006;67(6):309–12.
3. Coblation product brochure. Available at: https://www.smith-nephew.com/global/assets/pdf/products/surgical/sportsmedicine/08427f%20multi-electrode%20technology%20brochure.pdf. Accessed July 30, 2016.
4. Joshi H, Woodworth BA, Carney AS. Coblation for epistaxis management in patients with hereditary haemorrhagic telangiectasia: a multicentre case series. J Laryngol Otol 2011;125(11):1176–80.

5. Cavaliere M, Mottola G, Iemma M. Monopolar and bipolar radiofrequency thermal ablation of inferior turbinates. Otolaryngol Head Neck Surg 2007;137(2):256–63.

6. Gindros G, Kantas I, Balatsouras DG, et al. Comparison of ultrasound turbinate reduction, radiofrequency tissue ablation and submucosal cauterization in inferior turbinate hypertrophy. Eur Arch Otorhinolaryngol 2010;267(11):1727–33.

7. Sozansky J, Houser SM. Pathophysiology of empty nose syndrome. Laryngoscope 2015;125(1):70–4.

8. Berger G, Ophir D, Pitaro K, et al. Histopathological changes after coblation inferior turbinate reduction. Arch Otolaryngol Head Neck Surg 2008;134(8):819–23.

9. Hegazy HM, ElBadawey MR, Behery A. Inferior turbinate reduction; coblation versus microdebrider-a prospective, randomised study. Rhinology 2014;52(4): 306–14.

10. Liu C-M, Tan C-D, Lee F-P, et al. Microdebrider-assisted versus radiofrequency-assisted inferior turbinoplasty. Laryngoscope 2009;119(2):414–8.

11. Passali D, Loglisci M, Politi L, et al. Managing turbinate hypertrophy: coblation vs. radiofrequency treatment. Eur Arch Otorhinolaryngol 2016;273(6):1449–53.

12. Shah AN, Brewster D, Mitzen K, et al. Radiofrequency coblation versus intramural bipolar cautery for the treatment of inferior turbinate hypertrophy. Ann Otol Rhinol Laryngol 2015;124(9):691–7.

13. Jiang ZY, Pereira KD, Friedman NR, et al. Inferior turbinate surgery in children: a survey of practice patterns. Laryngoscope 2012;122(7):1620–3.

14. Tanna N, Im DD, Azhar H, et al. Inferior turbinoplasty during cosmetic rhinoplasty: techniques and trends. Ann Plast Surg 2014;72(1):5–8.

15. Eloy JA, Walker TJ, Casiano RR, et al. Effect of coblation polypectomy on estimated blood loss in endoscopic sinus surgery. Am J Rhinol Allergy 2009;23(5): 535–9.

16. Swibel-Rosenthal LH, Benninger MS, Stone CH, et al. Wound healing in the paranasal sinuses after Coblation, Part II: evaluation for endoscopic sinus surgery using a sheep model. Am J Rhinol Allergy 2010;24(6):464–6.

17. Swibel Rosenthal LH, Benninger MS, Stone CH, et al. Wound healing in the rabbit paranasal sinuses after Coblation: evaluation for use in endoscopic sinus surgery. Am J Rhinol Allergy 2009;23(3):360–3.

18. Kostrzewa JP, Sunde J, Riley KO, et al. Radiofrequency coblation decreases blood loss during endoscopic sinonasal and skull base tumor removal. ORL J Otorhinolaryngol Relat Spec 2010;72(1):38–43.

19. Athanasiadis T, Beule A, Embate J, et al. Standardized video-endoscopy and surgical field grading scale for endoscopic sinus surgery: a multi-centre study. Laryngoscope 2008;118(2):314–9.

20. Cannon DE, Poetker DM, Loehrl TA, et al. Use of coblation in resection of juvenile nasopharyngeal angiofibroma. Ann Otol Rhinol Laryngol 2013;122(6):353–7.

21. Ye L, Zhou X, Li J, et al. Coblation-assisted endonasal endoscopic resection of juvenile nasopharyngeal angiofibroma. J Laryngol Otol 2011;125(9):940–4.

22. Smith N, Riley KO, Woodworth BA. Endoscopic Coblator-assisted management of encephaloceles. Laryngoscope 2010;120(12):2535–9.

23. Gluckman JL, Portugal LG. Modified Young's procedure for refractory epistaxis due to hereditary hemorrhagic telangiectasia. Laryngoscope 1994;104(9): 1174–7.

24. Harvey RJ, Kanagalingam J, Lund VJ. The impact of septodermoplasty and potassium-titanyl-phosphate (KTP) laser therapy in the treatment of hereditary hemorrhagic telangiectasia-related epistaxis. Am J Rhinol 2008;22(2):182–7.

25. Ghaheri BA, Fong KJ, Hwang PH. The utility of bipolar electrocautery in hereditary hemorrhagic telangiectasia. Otolaryngol Head Neck Surg 2006;134(6): 1006–9.

26. Bublik M, Sargi Z, Casiano RR. Use of the microdebrider in selective excision of hereditary hemorrhagic telangiectasia: a new approach. Otolaryngol Head Neck Surg 2007;137(1):157–8.

27. Kim J-W, Kim HJ, Lee WH, et al. Comparative study for efficacy and safety of adenoidectomy according to the surgical method: a prospective multicenter study. PLoS One 2015;10(8):e0135304.

28. Thottam PJ, Christenson JR, Cohen DS, et al. The utility of common surgical instruments for pediatric adenotonsillectomy. Laryngoscope 2015;125(2):475–9.

29. Shah UK, Theroux Z, Shah GB, et al. Resource analysis of tonsillectomy in children. Laryngoscope 2014;124(5):1223–8.

Application of Ultrasonic Aspirators in Rhinology and Skull Base Surgery

Dominic Vernon, MD[a], Brian C. Lobo, MD[b],
Jonathan Y. Ting, MD, MS, MBA[a],*

KEYWORDS

- Ultrasonic aspirator • Piezosurgery • Endoscopic DCR • Turbinoplasty
- Skull base surgery

KEY POINTS

- Ultrasonic aspirators can safely be used in endoscopic sinus, orbital, and endonasal skull base surgery to safely remove soft tissue and bone.
- Size, length, and angle of handpiece and working tips can limit some endoscopic dissections.
- Integrated navigation is not available at this time on ultrasonic aspirators but would be a welcome addition. Moreover, they do not significantly alter either electromagnetic (EM) or optical guidance systems.
- Much like microdebriders, these must be used with great care around vital structures, with additional caution around the external nose and upper lip.

EVOLUTION OF THE ULTRASONIC ASPIRATOR

Ultrasonic aspirators (UAs) rely on the use of ultrasonic vibration to remove both mineralized and nonmineralized tissue. This phenomenon is possible due to the piezoelectric effect, first discovered by French physicists Jacques and Pierre Curie in 1880. The Curie brothers observed that applying pressure or mechanical stress to certain materials generated an external electric field due to shifting of positive and negative charges, thus converting mechanical energy to electrical energy. Equally fascinating is that the reverse is also true. Applying an external electric field to piezoelectric

Disclosures: The authors have no conflicting funding or financial interests to disclose.
[a] Department of Otolaryngology – Head and Neck Surgery, Indiana University School of Medicine, Indiana University, Fesler Hall, 1130 West Michigan Street, Suite 400, Indianapolis, IN 46202, USA; [b] Rhinology, Sinus & Endoscopic Skull Base Surgery, Department of Otolaryngology – Head and Neck Surgery, Cleveland Clinic Foundation, 9500 Euclid Avenue, Desk A-71, Cleveland, OH 44195, USA
* Corresponding author.
E-mail address: joting@iupui.edu

material causes rapid compression and expansion of the material and creates ultrasonic oscillations. Harnessing this inverse piezoelectric effect is the foundation of UAs.[1-3] Although the Curie brothers demonstrated this effect using natural quartz and topaz, the overall piezoelectric effect of naturally occurring materials is relatively subtle. The development of synthetic ceramics with more powerful piezoelectric properties led to several practical applications, from simple devices, such as the cigarette lighter, to more complex medical devices, such as ultrasonic transducers and UAs.[1,2]

Using ultrasonic energy to cut bone or tissue is not new to medicine. Before the development of piezosurgery using the modern UA, the use of ultrasonic energy to cut dental tissue was described as early as 1953.[4] Ultrasonic aspiration was used to remove gingival plaques and assist in performing procedures such as root canals.[5] The harmonic scalpel, used to ligate and seal soft tissue, has been in use for the past few decades. The concept of the modern UA for what is described as piezosurgery is credited to Tomaso Vercellotti, who modified the existing technology to be more powerful and more precise.

As power and precision advanced, use of ultrasonic bone aspirators exploded in the fields of dentistry and oral maxillofacial surgery, in which ultrasonic technology was already in use. For the past 2 decades, this technology has been used for dental implant placement, Le Fort I osteotomies for midface deformities, and sagittal split osteotomies.[4,6] More recently, use of this technology by the otolaryngologic community has increased in a variety of neurotologic procedures, as well as rhinoplasty and medialization laryngoplasty.[7]

HOW THE TECHNOLOGY WORKS

As previously described, the modern UA relies on precise transformation of electrical energy to mechanical energy. The aspirator handpiece functions as the piezoelectric device, amplifying and transmitting vibrations to a variety of tips. The tips often have special coatings, including titanium and diamonds (**Fig. 1**). The frequency of device vibration can be adjusted but is most often set between 25 and 30 kHz. This is significant because it gives these devices the unique advantage of cutting mineralized bony tissue while minimizing damage to other soft tissue. These frequencies produce movements ranging from 60 to 210 μm, which cut bone but do little damage to soft tissue. Cutting soft tissue requires a frequency higher than 50 kHz, such as that seen with the

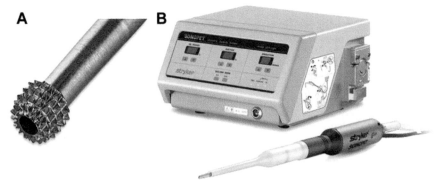

Fig. 1. Stryker Sonopet ultrasonic aspirator equipment. (*A*) Tip for ultrasonic aspirator. (*B*) Console and handpiece with integrated suction and irrigation. (*Courtesy of* Stryker, Kalamazoo, MI; with permission.)

use of the harmonic scalpel.[1-3] It is important to note that the tips designed for bony use can still damage surrounding tissues because at least 1 in vivo study has demonstrated the capability of functional damage to nerves on direct exposure to the device.[8] However, this was seen with prolonged direct contact on the nerve, a situation avoidable with meticulous dissection.

Although UAs rely on vibration to remove tissue, the actual mechanism of tissue removal is properly described as cavitation. The high-frequency oscillations serve to break down hydrogen bonds, causing the denaturation of proteins in tissue. Tissue is subsequently emulsified by the formation of vapor bubbles, and this slurry is quickly washed away by the accompanying irrigation. An irrigation system is often contained within the handpiece to cool bone as the device cuts and also to clear the surgical field and maintain visualization.[1-3]

In addition to its soft tissue–sparing properties, piezosurgery has also demonstrated more favorable bone healing after surgery compared with the use of some other more conventional methods. Histologic studies have demonstrated that over the course of the first 90 days of bone healing, surgical sites using piezosurgery have increased osteoblastic activity and an overall greater rate of healing when compared with the mechanical burr. Cellular reorganization and osteoid formation may occur as early as 3 days postpiezosurgery.[9] Vercellotti and colleagues[10] used an animal model to investigate levels of bone healing in the UA, carbide burr, and diamond burr. As early as 2 weeks after ostectomy, piezosurgery sites demonstrated an increase in bone compared with baseline levels, whereas both burrs demonstrated an overall loss in bone stock. This trend was seen at postoperative day 56 as well.

This favorable osseous response in piezosurgery may be due to decreased thermal energy transmitted to bone, resulting in less trauma overall to surrounding bony and soft tissues. Of note, drilled surgical sites show an increased level of inflammatory cells compared with sites removed with UAs. Additionally, surgical sites using UAs seem to have earlier increases in favorable cytokines and growth factors, such as BMP-4 (bone morphogenetic protein) and TGF-beta2 (transforming growth factor). For these reasons, there has been increased interest in using piezosurgery to harvest bone chips and grafts.[11-13]

SURGICAL TECHNIQUE

It should be noted that the technique of an UA in surgery to remove bone differs from more conventional saws or drills. Unlike conventional instruments, which require application of significant pressure to perform cuts, the UA only requires a minimal amount of pressure. The instruments should glide firmly over the area of intended bony removal because undue pressure can actually be counterproductive, slowing the tip vibration and inhibiting the irrigation system from effectively cooling the target tissue. Applying a large amount of pressure can cause excessive heat generation and prevent the UA from functioning optimally. The surgeon should be aware of these principles when operating the UA. Firm but light movement over the bone allows efficient and precise removal with minimal generation of heat.[1-3]

The benefits of the UA are numerous. Few instruments allow for the selective removal of bone with minimal trauma to adjacent soft tissues. Additionally, the lack of a spinning bit allows for increased precision in the takedown of osseous structures, reducing the risk of slipping or skipping as seen with more conventional spinning drill bits (**Table 1** for a comparison of powered otolaryngology instruments.). The utility of these instruments was not lost to the otolaryngologist, and the field has already demonstrated the use of the harmonic oscillator in many subspecialties, including

Table 1
Comparison of powered otolaryngology instruments

	Ultrasonic Aspirator	High-Speed Drill	Microdebrider
Powered or manual	Powered	Powered	Powered
Mechanism of tissue removal	Cavitation via ultrasonic vibrations	Mechanical via drill burrs	Mechanical via rotating blades
Suction capability	Yes	No	Yes
Self-irrigating	Yes	Yes	Yes
Heat generation	Mild	Moderate-high	Minimal
Navigation capability	Yes[a]	Yes[a]	Yes
Selective tissue removal	Yes[b]	No	No

[a] May be adapted for navigation with existing systems but navigation not built into device.
[b] Ultrasonic frequencies set to 25 to 30 kHz selectivity cavitate mineralized tissue are relatively atraumatic to soft tissue structures.

facial plastics, otology, and laryngology. Rhinology is no exception, with the first endoscopic use described in 2008 by Antisdel and colleagues[14] for endoscopic dacryocystorhinostomy (E-DCR). Since that time, the role of the UA has continued to expand in endoscopic sinus surgery and endoscopic skull base surgery.[15]

INFERIOR TURBINOPLASTY AND SEPTOPLASTY

Although several surgical techniques are available for addressing inferior turbinate hypertrophy, some surgeons now advocate the use of the UA for this purpose. In 2010, Greywoode and colleagues[16] first described using ultrasonic aspiration turbinoplasty in a series of 81 subjects. In this technique, the inferior turbinate is medialized and an incision is made in the head of the inferior turbinate down to the level of the bone. Subperiosteal dissection to elevate tissue off the bony turbinate is then performed and an UA is used to remove the conchal bone before lateralization of the turbinate at the completion of the procedure. No complications relating to the turbinoplasty procedure were reported in the population of 81 subjects. A small subset of 7 subjects completing preoperative and postoperative Nasal Obstruction Symptom Evaluation (NOSE) forms showed a significant decrease in nasal obstructive symptoms. However, the overall assessment of the procedure's effectiveness is limited because all subjects also underwent some form of additional nasal surgery at the time of the turbinoplasty, including rhinoplasty, septoplasty, functional endoscopic sinus surgery, or dacryocystorhinostomy (DCR).

Kim and colleagues[17] recently published the results of a study of 30 subjects in which an UA was used to perform a portion of septoturbinoplasty. The investigators described the increased precision of the instrument for use in removing bony spurs, deviated maxillary crests, and the bony septum compared with more conventional methods such as the osteotome. The investigators noted the UA has the benefit of sparing mucosal injury to mucoperichondrial flaps during removal of the bony septum. The NOSE scale was used preoperatively and postoperatively in all subjects in this particular study, and a significant decrease in symptoms of nasal obstruction was noted. Acoustic rhinometry was used as an objective measure of nasal patency preoperatively and postoperatively, with significant improvements in nasal cross-sectional area noted after surgery. No complications were reported with the use of ultrasonic aspiration. It must be noted that the cartilaginous septum was removed conventionally and, in most subjects, the turbinate microdebrider was used in addition to the UA for turbinate soft tissue reduction.

Although it seems clear from preliminary studies that the UA is a safe adjunctive tool for bony work, evidence regarding increased benefit over traditional techniques is lacking. Its primary advantages come from its ability to spare mucosal tissue in the limited workspace environment of both turbinoplasty and septoplasty. In select patients with severe bony septal deviations or primarily bony turbinate hypertrophy, the aspirator would be a useful available adjunct. However, its use remains limited in patients with primarily cartilaginous deflections or soft tissue turbinate hypertrophy.

ENDOSCOPIC DACRYOCYSTORHINOSTOMY

DCR, a procedure used for relief of nasolacrimal duct obstruction, required an external approach before the use of the endoscope. Since then, the endoscopic approach has become the preferred approach for many surgeons. E-DCR lends itself well to the application of the UA for multiple reasons. The surgery is confined to a small working area intimately associated with the middle turbinate and the orbital contents, where even minor mucosal damage can have dire consequences. In addition, the bone overlying the lacrimal sac is fairly thick, which in the past required removal with powered instruments, such as drills, or manually using curettes or rongeurs. The inherent danger in using these devices is the possibility of injury to the underlying lacrimal sac or nearby mucosa, which can result in scarring and resultant failure. The UA, with its mucosal-sparing properties, offers a safe and efficient means of bone removal in this procedure.

The first use of the UA in E-DCR was described by Antisdel and colleagues,[14] who reported the results of 12 subjects (total of 16 procedures) undergoing the procedure. The investigators reported the ease of the device in creating the bony rhinostomy, and reported no injuries to the lacrimal sac in any cases. Additionally, even with accidental or purposeful movement over nearby mucosa, no damage was noted. Postoperative results were favorable. With a mean follow-up of 20 months, all subjects had resolution of their symptoms. Additionally, patency was confirmed with the use of fluorescein dye in all subjects.

Salami and colleagues[18] described similar results in a slightly larger series of 20 subjects all undergoing E-DCR with UA. After the aspirator was used to completely expose the lacrimal sac by removing all overlying maxillary bone, all subjects were seen at 12 months postoperatively. Strict definitions of failure were outlined for the study, which included no improvement of symptoms, nasal endoscopy showing obstruction of the ostium by scarring or granulation, obstruction by dacryoscintigraphy, or negative functional endoscopic dye test. No postoperative failures were reported by the investigators in this series of 20 subjects. As previously reviewed, histologic studies suggest that the UA is superior in terms of promoting bone healing compared with more conventional methods. The investigators feel this superior healing may have a benefit in terms of reducing the risk of restenosis in E-DCR.

Comparison of E-DCR by UA and powered microdrill was performed by Steele and colleagues[19] in a retrospective review. Sixty-three subjects were included in the study, with 29 undergoing E-DCR with the conventional drill and 34 undergoing ultrasonic bone aspirator E-DCR. Although the ultrasonic procedure had a slightly higher success rate at 94.1% (86.2% success rate was seen for the microdrill), no statistical significance was noted. Failure of the ultrasonic procedure was seen in 2 subjects and was related to scarring at the neo-ostium. No other complications were reported in either group. These success rates are slightly higher than those of an earlier retrospective study involving 123 subjects undergoing E-DCR, in which success rates were 81.3% in subjects not undergoing ultrasonic E-DCR and 79.7% in those undergoing ultrasonic E-DCR.[20] Again, no statistically significant difference between groups was noted, and no major complications were reported.

More recently, a prospective trial was performed comparing the surgical time of E-DCR with a mechanical drill to E-DCR using the UA. Fifty-five subjects were included, 29 in the drill groups and 26 in the piezosurgery group. No significant difference in operative time was noted (3.71 min vs 4.12 min, $P = .17$). One minor complication was noted in the piezosurgery group: superficial burns to the nasal vestibule occurred when irrigation malfunctioned within the ultrasonic handpiece. However, this healed without any residual scarring. The study did not include any postoperative follow-up, so the long-term patency rates between the 2 methods could not be assessed.[21]

There are more robust data for the use of ultrasonic bone aspiration for E-DCR than any other rhinology procedure, largely because it is the earliest reported use of this technology in the rhinologic literature. Studies indicate a strong safety profile, and multiple retrospective reviews have confirmed success rates that are equivalent to previous methods such the mechanical burr. Additionally, the benefits of using an UA in E-DCR are multifold. The device allows for precise control in a tight surgical window and is extremely forgiving around surrounding soft tissue structures. Familiarity with the device would be essential to any rhinologist planning to perform such procedures.

SKULL BASE SURGERY

Advances in visualization and instrumentation have expanded the role of the rhinologist in the past 3 decades. Increased collaboration with neurosurgical colleagues has led to endoscopic approaches for intracranial lesions of the central skull base. The neurosurgeon is no stranger to ultrasonic aspiration technology, with the earliest clinical use reported by Flamm and colleagues[22] years before its introduction to otolaryngology. Ultrasonic aspiration has been used in the intracapsular resection of firm intracranial tumors, as well as in the evacuation of large intraventricular hematomas via neuroendoscopy, sparing patients open surgery.[23,24] With an increasing number of endoscopic skull base approaches being used, piezosurgery continues to find new applications in otolaryngology and neurosurgery.

The most common endoscopic skull base approach is the transsphenoidal approach for resection of pituitary tumors. This approach can require removing a considerable amount of bone during the posterior septectomy and removal of sphenoid rostrum and septae. Traditionally, this approach is done using cold steel instruments such as Kerrison rongeurs; through-cuts; backbiters; and, more recently, endoscopic skull base drills. With the recent advent of UAs in otolaryngology, there has been increased interest in applying this technology to the transsphenoidal approach (**Figs. 2–4**). The use of the aspirator for the removal of more firm pituitary tumors has also been described.[24,25]

A recent cadaveric study investigated the feasibility of using piezosurgery to create bone flaps during the transsphenoidal approach.[26] The creation of bone flaps using an endoscopic approach can be difficult, particularly with nonpowered instruments. Using an UA, Tomazic and colleagues[26] were able to easily create craniotomies of 3 to 5 cm within the sellar floor, tuberculum sellae, and planum sphenoidale. The bone flaps were created without fracturing and could be easily reimplanted.

One of the largest studies investigating the use of the UA in anterior skull base surgery is a randomized controlled trial comparing the aspirator to traditional cold steel

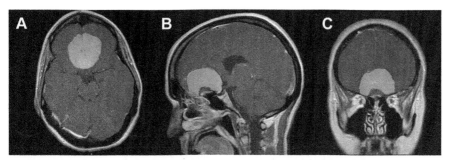

Fig. 2. Olfactory groove meningioma. Preoperative contrasted MRI images. (*A*) Axial image. (*B*) Sagittal image. (*C*) Coronal image.

instruments in the transsphenoidal approach.[24] Both operative time and blood loss were tracked in 130 subjects undergoing transsphenoidal approaches for pituitary lesions. The subjects were randomized to either a traditional approach with nonpowered instruments or an approach using the aspirator for all bony removal. A significant reduction in operating time was seen in the UA group. The average operative time was 9.4 minutes faster (31.92 + 3.04 min vs 41.32 + 2.75 min, $P<.0001$). Blood loss was also significantly lowered (16.5 + 5.37 mL vs 22.57 + 3.09 mL, $P<.0001$). No adverse events or complications were reported related to the use new technology.

This study also raised concerns regarding cost of UA technology. The device was shown to be a safe and efficient means of bone removal. However, the reduction in blood loss was clinically negligible, and the reduction in operating time did not translate to a reduction in cost, especially when taking into consideration the price of the UA equipment. The UA ultimately remains a useful tool in the skillset of the endoscopic skull base surgeon, though its use may be more suited to more challenging cases requiring precise removal of bone. Undoubtedly, its role will continue to expand as the technology continues to improve and becomes even more readily available.

FUNCTIONAL ENDOSCOPIC SINUS SURGERY

Several investigators have reported on the usefulness of piezosurgery in select endoscopic sinus surgery cases, in particular the removal of bony tumors such as

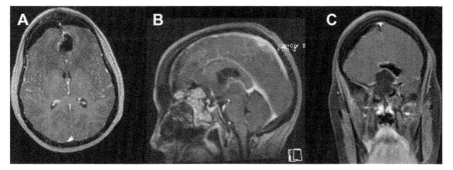

Fig. 3. Olfactory groove meningioma. Postoperative contrasted MRI images. Resection was carried out via an endoscopic approach with the ultrasonic aspirator. (*A*) Axial image. (*B*) Sagittal image. (*C*) Coronal image.

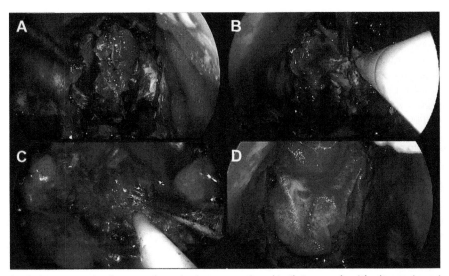

Fig. 4. Intraoperative images of meningioma resection. (*A–C*) Approach with ultrasonic aspirator for removal of bony tissue. (*D*) Duragen (Integra LifeSciences, Plainsboro, NJ) underlay placed within skull base defect.

osteomas. Pagella and colleagues[27] describe the first case of endoscopic osteoma removal using the UA in a case of a frontoethmoidal osteoma. A conventional Draf IIa procedure was used for exposure before takedown with an angled UA under visualization with a 70° endoscope. Gotlib and colleagues[28] described a similar approach for a type IV frontal osteoma, first performing a Draf IIb for exposure using conventional instruments. This case described removal of both frontal beak and intersinus septum remnants using both drills and piezosurgery. The frontal osteoma was removed with the use of the UA alone. No complications were reported in either case. Both investigators comment on the usefulness of the device in terms of sparing soft tissue structures. Theoretically, the risk of cerebrospinal fluid leak in these complicated cases is lower if using ultrasonic technology because the risk of direct damage to the dura is minimized.

Increasing familiarity with piezosurgery has led to some use of the device in more routine endoscopic sinus surgery. Mancini and colleagues[29] describe a small case series in which piezosurgery was used for submucosal maxillary antrostomy, addressing concha bullosa, and even performing a submucosal removal of the ethmoid bulla. The UA has also been touted as a useful adjunct in revision endoscopic cases, particularly in the case of patients with osteoneogenesis near crucial structures. Bolger[30] describes the utility of the device in removing hard bone adjacent to the orbit or skull base in 14 revision cases and reported no complications related to its use.

SUMMARY

Technological advances will continue to drive rhinology forward. Just as microdebriders were adapted for rhinologic use from orthopedic surgery, the UA, once a favored tool of dental surgeons and dentists, has seen a recent expansion in use by rhinologists. The efficacy of this technology in E-DCR is well documented and can be considered equivalent to standard powered techniques both in terms of operative time and success rates. Increasing interest has been shown in septoturbinoplasty, in which precise bony removal is necessary to mucosal preservation, and applications in central skull base surgery have shown promise with respect to reduced blood loss and operative time, and decreased risk of damage to critical structures. The benefits of the technology may extend to revision endoscopic sinus surgery, in which it may be necessary to remove thick osteitic bone against the orbit or skull base. The UA is an extremely versatile instrument, and it would be useful for any rhinologist to have a working knowledge of this technology. Its unique ability to remove bone while sparing soft tissue structures make it ideal for the endoscopic surgeon, whose primary goal is often to preserve as much functional mucosa as possible. It is important, however, to note the cost of the technology with the significant attention paid to ballooning health care costs, as well as the possibility for soft tissue injury due to overheating.

REFERENCES

1. Pavlikova G, Foltan R, Hanzelka T, et al. Piezosurgery in oral and maxillofacial surgery. Int J Oral Maxillofac Surg 2011;40:451–7.
2. Labanca M, Azzola F, Vinci R, et al. Piezoelectric surgery: twenty years of use. Br J Oral Maxillofac Surg 2000;38:530–2.
3. Bruggers S, Sindwani R. Evolving trends in powered endoscopic sinus surgery. Otolaryngol Clin North Am 2009;42:789–98.
4. Catuna MC. Sonic surgery. Ann Dent 1953;12:100.
5. Eggers G, Klein J, Blank J, et al. Piezosurgery: an ultrasound device for cutting bone and its use and limitations in maxillofacial surgery. Br J Oral Maxillofac Surg 2004;42:451–3.
6. Chen YL, Chang H, Chiang Y, et al. Application and development of ultrasonics in dentistry. J Formos Med Assoc 2013;112:659–65.
7. Salami A, Massimo D, Proto E, et al. Piezosurgery in otologic surgery: Four years of experience. Otolaryngol Head Neck Surg 2009;140:412–8.
8. Schareren S, Jaquiery C, Heberer M, et al. Assessment of nerve damage using a novel ultrasonic device for bone cutting. J Oral Maxillofac Surg 2008;66:593–6.
9. Horton JE, Tarpley TM, Wood LD. The healing of surgical defects in alveolar bone produced with ultrasonic instrumentation, chisel, and rotary bur. Oral Surg Oral Med Oral Pathol 1975;39:536–46.
10. Vercellotti T, Nevins ML, Kim DM, et al. Osseous response following respective therapy with piezosurgery. Int J Periodontics Restorative Dent 2005;25:543–9.
11. Preti G, Martinasso G, Peirone B, et al. Cytokines and growth factors involved in the osseointegration of oral titanium implants positioned using piezoelectric bone surgery versus a drill technique: a pilot study in minipigs. J Periodontol 2007;78: 716–22.
12. Chiriac G, Herten M, Schwarz F, et al. Autogenous bone chips: influence of a new piezoelectric device (Piezosurgery) on chip morphology, cell viability and differentiation. J Clin Periodontol 2005;32:994–9.
13. Berengo M, Bacci C, Sartori M, et al. Histomorphometric evaluation of bone grafts harvested by different methods. Minerva Stomatol 2006;55:189–98.
14. Antisdel JL, Kadze MS, Sindwani R. Application of ultrasonic aspirators to endoscopic dacryocystorhinostomy. Otolaryngol Head Neck Surg 2009;139:586–8.
15. Ye T, Zhou B. Update on surgical management of adult inferior turbinate hypertrophy. Curr Opin Otolaryngol Head Neck Surg 2015;23:29–33.
16. Greywoode JD, Van Abel K, Pribitkin EA. Ultrasonic bone aspirator turbinoplasty: a novel approach for management of inferior turbinate hypertrophy. Laryngoscope 2010;120:S239.

17. Kim JY, Choi G, Kwon JH. The application of an ultrasonic bone aspirator for sep-toturbinoplasty. J Craniofac Surg 2015;26:893–6.

18. Salami A, Dellepiane M, Salzano FA, et al. Piezosurgery in endoscopic dacryo-cystorhinostomy. Otolaryngol Head Neck Surg 2009;140:264–6.

19. Steele T, Wilson M, Strong B. Ultrasonic bone aspirator assisted endoscopic da-cryocystorhinostomy. Am J Otolaryngol Head Neck Surg 2016;37:202–6.

20. Murchison AP, Pribitkin EA, Rosen MR, et al. The ultrasonic bone aspirator in transnasal endoscopic dacryocystorhinostomy. Ophthal Plast Reconstr Surg 2013;20:24–9.

21. Ali MJ, Ganguly A, Ali MH, et al. Time taken for superior osteotomy in primary powered endoscopic dacryocystorhinostomy: is there a difference between an ultrasonic aspirator and a mechanical burr? Int Forum Allergy Rhinol 2015;5: 764–7.

22. Flamm E, Ransohoff J, Wuchinich D, et al. Preliminary experience with ultrasonic aspiration in neurosurgery. Congress Neurol Surgeons 1978;2:240–5.

23. Oka K, Go Y, Yamamoto M, et al. Experience with an ultrasonic aspirator in neuro-endoscopy. Minim Invasive Neurosurg 1999;42:32–4.

24. Baddour HM, Lupa MD, Patel ZM. Comparing use of the Sonopet ultrasonic bone aspirator to traditional instrumentation during the endoscopic transsphenodial approach in pituitary tumor resection. Int Forum Allergy Rhinol 2013;3:588–91.

25. Zador Z, Gnanalingham K. Endoscopic transnasal approach to the pituitary – oper-ative techniques and nuances. Br J Neurosurg 2013;27:718–26.

26. Tomazic PV, Gellner V, Koele W, et al. Feasibility of piezoelectric endoscopic transsphenoidal craniotomy: a cadaveric study. Biomed Res Int 2014;2014: 341876.

27. Pagella F, Giourgos G, Matti E, et al. Removal of a fronto-ethmoidal osteoma us-ing the sonopet omni ultrasonic bone curette: first impressions. Laryngoscope 2008;118:307–9.

28. Gotlib T, Niemczyk K. Transnasal endoscopic piezoelectric-assisted removal of frontal sinus osteoma. Laryngoscope 2013;123:588–90.

29. Mancini G, Buonaccorsi S, Reale G, et al. Application of piezoelectric device in endoscopic sinus surgery. J Craniofac Surg 2012;23:1736–40.

30. Bolger WE. Piezoelectric surgical device in endoscopic sinus surgery: an initial clinical experience. Ann Otol Rhinol Laryngol 2009;118:621–4.

Next-Generation Surgical Navigation Systems in Sinus and Skull Base Surgery

Martin J. Citardi, MD*, William Yao, MD, Amber Luong, MD, PhD

KEYWORDS

- Surgical navigation • Endoscopic sinus surgery • Computer-aided surgery
- Augmented reality • Microsensors

KEY POINTS

- Surgical navigation, also known as image-guided surgery, has been widely adopted for endoscopic sinus and skull base surgery because most surgeons find the technology useful for facilitating procedures of moderate-to-high complexity.
- For surgical navigation to be useful, the accuracy (more formally known as target registration error [TRE]) must be 2 mm or better. Commercially available systems often achieve TRE of 1.5 to 2.0 mm but, too often, TRE is greater than 2.0 mm. For this reason, surgeons cannot completely trust the technology.
- A next-generation surgical navigation system should strive for a TRE of 1.0 to 1.5 mm (or even 0.5–1.0 mm) with a "tight" error range, levels that will push technical boundaries. Innovations in hardware and software will be necessary to achieve this transformation.
- Augmented reality technology (which provides additional visual cues or annotations to real-world images) can also be incorporated into surgical navigation.
- Microsensors for electromagnetic tracking systems will open new opportunities for surgical navigation, with unique applications for balloon catheter placement and targeted drug delivery.

INTRODUCTION

Since the early 1990s, surgical navigation has emerged as a critical tool during the era of endoscopic surgery of the paranasal sinuses and adjacent skull base. From its inception, surgical navigation (also known as image-guided surgery, or IGS)

Conflicts of Interest: M.J. Citardi serves as a consultant for Acclarent (Irvine, CA), Biosense Webster (Haifa, Israel), Medical Metrics (Houston, TX) and Medtronic (Jacksonville, FL). A. Luong serves as a consultant for 480 Biomedical (Watertown, MA). The Department receives research funds from Intersect ENT (Menlo Park, CA) and Allakos (San Carlos, CA).
Department of Otorhinolaryngology–Head and Neck Surgery, McGovern Medical School, The University of Texas Health Science Center at Houston, 6431 Fannin Street, MSB 5.036, Houston, TX 77030, USA
* Corresponding author.
E-mail address: martin.j.citardi@uth.tmc.edu

provided a way for surgeons to track an instrument tip relative to the preoperative imaging data set. Through successive iterations of the hardware and software, the technology has become more robust and user-friendliness has improved dramatically; yet, the core features have remained essentially unchanged. In fact, today's systems greatly resemble first-generation systems, which is a remarkable fact in light of the technological progress of related devices and software over the past 20 years. Recently, new surgical navigation systems have been introduced into the United States and global markets, and companies are developing innovative surgical navigation technology, which is likely to be commercially released relatively soon. Thus, it is an opportune time to assess current technology trends.

CURRENT STATE OF THE ART

Surgeon surveys performed over the past decade suggest greater availability of surgical navigation technology in most ear, nose, and throat (ENT) operating rooms in the United States and confirm that a large number of sinus surgeons are comfortable with the technology, especially for more advanced sinus cases.[1–3] These survey data are consistent with the theme of wide-spread surgeon acceptance across all types of operating room settings. In 2002, the American Academy of Otolaryngology—Head and Neck Surgery first issued its position statement on computer-aided surgery, an inclusive term that includes surgical navigation, and has periodically updated it.[4] This statement emphasizes that, although use of the technology is at the discretion of the operating surgeon, the technology should not be deemed experimental and has wide indications, including revision sinus surgery, skull base surgery, frontal sinus surgery, and so forth.

Obviously surgeons choose to use surgical navigations to achieve better clinical outcomes. Data that prove this point are relatively sparse. At least 2 studies suggest that surgical navigation is associated with lower intraoperative blood loss.[5,6] One study did demonstrate better Rhinosinusitis Outcome Measure (RSOM)-31 scores in patients whose endoscopic sinus surgery (ESS) was performed with surgical navigation.[7] A reduction in revision surgery has been associated with the use of surgical navigation.[8] However, other studies tried to show similar advantages and were not successful in proving this point.[9–12]

Anecdotally, surgeons report that surgical navigation has a positive influence on the performance of the surgical procedure. Numerous studies suggest that surgical navigation actually may lengthen the procedure,[6,13–16] but that is not the point. In an early retrospective study, Reardon[13] showed comparable complication rates in cohorts of patients whose sinus surgery was performed with and without surgical navigation, although the subjects in whom surgical navigation was used tended to have more sinuses entered. This suggests that the surgeon's comfort zone expanded through the use of surgical navigation. In a novel study, Strauss and colleagues[17] assessed the impact of surgical navigation by capturing the intraoperative change of surgical strategy associated with the application of the navigation device. In approximately, 50% of individual localizations, the use of the technology resulted in a change in surgical strategy. This study corroborates the reports of almost all surgeons who use surgical navigation and find it distinctly helpful.

From the time of its introduction, surgical navigation held the promise of a reduction in complication rates. In practice, it has been difficult to confirm this intuitive supposition. Some studies have shown no reduction in complications.[18,19] In a retrospective review, Fried and colleagues[5] noted a lower complication rate in subjects whose ESS was performed with navigation. This was later corroborated in a similar study.[16] In fact, Ramakrishnan and colleagues[19] published a systematic review in 2013 and concluded that the published literature does not support either reduced complications or better outcomes with surgical navigation. It should be kept in mind that demonstrating such advantages would require a prospective study of 35,000 subjects,[20] which is a major hurdle for something that already garnered mainstream acceptance. Most recently, Dalgorf and colleagues[21] did another major meta-analysis that seems to finally confirm that surgical navigation is associated with fewer major and minor complications.

Two types of instrument tracking systems have been used for surgical navigation. Optical systems rely on a camera array to triangulate the position of light-emitting diodes or reflective spheres attached to instruments, whereas in an electromagnetic (EM) navigation, copper coils attached to instruments act as sensors that detect changes in an EM field sustained by the system's dedicated emitter. In theory, optical systems are viewed as more reliable for measuring positions because they are not subject to EM field distortions that produce inaccuracies for instrument tracking. The major drawback for any optical system is the requirement for maintaining a line-of-sight between the instrument tracker and the camera array. EM systems avoid this issue and thus are preferred by most surgeons. Both optical and EM systems seem to generate comparable accuracy in the actual operating room.[22] This suggests that surgical navigation performance represents a wide variety of factors, beyond the intrinsic capacity to sense and measure instrument position.

LIMITATIONS OF CURRENT SYSTEMS

Almost every publication, presentation, and discussion on surgical navigation includes the warning that, although surgical navigation may be viewed as a critically important piece of technology, surgeons should be loath to depend on it. In essence, surgeons are advised to trust their surgical judgment, not technology. The rationale for this posture is obvious: despite the wealth of useful information provided by surgical navigation, which many surgeons have come to use routinely, the technology has an unacceptable failure rate. Specifically, it can be remarkably accurate in many instances and then give a spurious localization in a pattern that seems random. If the surgeon does not recognize the false localization, the results could be catastrophic. For this reason, the threshold for dismissing a questionable localization is very low, undermining the utility of navigation.

This critical observation must be placed in the context of the common understanding about human perception, which can be easily deceived, deliberately or inadvertently. Surgeons are often compared with pilots and aircraft processes are popular in many operating rooms. In fact, the surgical checklist is based on the positive experiences of the aerospace industry, in which checklists have led to dramatic increases in safety. Interestingly, pilots are always advised to trust their instruments, a posture that is directly opposite to approach of surgeons in regard to surgical navigation. Ultimately, this reflects a failure of surgical navigation to completely fulfill its initial promises.

A complete discussion of registration processes and registration error theory is beyond the scope of this article but it will be useful to summarize clinically achievable surgical navigation accuracy (more accurately termed target registration error [TRE]).[23] The general consensus is that TRE should be 2 mm or less for surgical navigation to be useful.[24] Reported mean TRE values in published reports range from 1.5 mm to 2.3 mm.[23] Some of the published data on TRE are in cadaveric models or in dry laboratories; therefore, these reports may not represent what is achievable in the real world. Furthermore, it must be remembered that each TRE is reported as a mean plus a standard deviation; therefore, there is a range of values and it is likely that some of the range is above the critical 2 mm level established as the highest clinically acceptable TRE. Finally, the frequency distribution of TRE values is positively skewed. For this reason, some TRE values will be 2 or more times greater than the stated mean value. The bottom line is that current registration protocols work well quite often but the prevalence of high TRE (ie, inaccurate surgical navigation) is too great for surgeons to rely on navigation in the same way that pilots rely on instruments.

Current systems have other limitations. Most of the systems are bulky and require a dedicated tower just for the navigation system. In the current shift of procedures to the office setting, this setting requires equipment with a small form factor, a physical parameter that had been a relative nonissue in the traditional operating room environment. Commonly, navigation systems have a separate monitor positioned to the side of the monitor that projects the endoscopic image. This arrangement offers poor ergonomics because the surgeon must constantly redirect his or her eyes and/or position his or her head to see the relevant visual information. In practice, this limits the use of the navigation system because the surgeon will tend to favor the endoscopic images.

Early in the era of surgical navigation, it was proposed that the localization information provided through surgical navigation should be directly integrated into the intraoperative planning and execution.[25] In practice, current surgical navigation technology falls short on this promise.

RETHINKING REGISTRATION

Early in the era of surgical navigation, some surgeons spoke erroneously about submillimetric accuracy. In fact, certain physical limitations make achieving a TRE of 1 mm extremely difficult. The best case TRE of a specific platform is a combination of 3 distinct and independent factors. First, the ability of the system to sense instrument position generates some error. Fortunately, this can be less than 1 mm on commercially available hardware but it can never be zero. Second, the quality of the imaging sets the lower limit. Conventional computed tomography (CT) produced imaging data at a slice thickness of as little as 0.5 mm. Although cone-beam CT scans offer even thinner slices, the resultant images do not provide the same crisp details of the bony anatomy. Thus, the lower limit for TRE is at least 0.5 mm using the best, commercially available CT scanners. Third, the registration process of mapping corresponding points from the patient to the imaging data set introduces additional error.

A TRE of 2.0 mm is clinically acceptable but any value more than 2.0 mm adversely affects the utility of the navigation information. Today, surgical navigation platforms produce mean TREs in the 1.5 to 2.0 mm range (ie, the best-case, real-world scenario). The next immediate goal for a next-generation surgical navigation platform would be to move TRE to 1.0 to 1.5 mm or, ideally, to 0.6 to 1.0 mm. A supplementary goal would be to eliminate or reduce the positive skew in the frequency distribution of TRE values. A dramatic stretch of current technical capabilities would be required to attain these goals.

In recent years, 2 novel approaches to contour-based registration have been introduced. Stryker PROFESS Navigation (Stryker, Kalamazoo, MI, USA) features pattern recognition optics for registration.[26] In this system, stickers with specific graphic markers are placed on the patient's nose, forehead, and cheeks at the beginning of surgery; these markers serve to define the contour. The tracking system is optical and the camera is incorporated into the instrument, not an overhead array. The camera on the instrument reads the position of contour for registration and actual navigation. The need to maintain line-of-sight is a major disadvantage of this approach. Another alternative for registration is the use of a photograph for registration purposes. The Tracey application (not commercially available in the United States as of the date of this publication), part of Fiagon Surgical Navigation (Fiagon, Berlin, Germany) incorporates a tablet computer for the picture, which is then uploaded to the main computer for calculating the registration.[27] In theory, photoregistration should be more accurate than contour-based registration because photoregistration collects many more fiducial points than the typical 200 to 500 points used for contour-based registration.

Because bone always would provide the optimal substrate for registration (rather than skin or soft tissue, which is deformable), registration protocols that incorporate fiducial points for bony landmarks are ideal. Bone-anchored fiducial makers, which are screws that are attached to the patient's skull, do tend to provide better TRE than contour-based registration protocols; however, this is not a clinically acceptable solution for rhinology procedures. In fact, even the bone-anchored markers tend to loosen and thus are suboptimal. An alternative approach would be to register to the bony contour of maxillofacial skeleton and cranial vault. In theory, an ultrasound-based probe would allow quick identification of hundreds (or even thousands) of points on the bone beneath the skin and provide data for robust, contour-based algorithm. Regrettably, such a technology has not been developed.

Smaller but still meaningful improvements in TRE may be achieved by adding additional points to the registration cloud from deep within the surgical field. It is important to remember that for contour-based registration (or for paired-point registration with anatomic landmarks) the fiducial points for surgical navigation are from the face. Picking up additional points from the sphenoid face or elsewhere may optimize the initial registration. Fiagon Surgical Navigation has an "Improve" tool intended to map points along the floor of the nose and lateral nasal wall. Karl Storz ENT Navigation Software 5.6.0 (Karl Storz, Tuttlingen, Germany) offers a similar software through which a point at the sphenoid may be incorporated into the fiducial point data set.[28]

Finally, it must be remembered that TRE that can be achieved in the clinical realm is the result of a complex interaction of many inter-related factors. Certainly, the software routines that perform the registration calculation, which are essentially algorithms that find the best fit between the fiducial points and the corresponding points in the imaging data, may be further optimized. Instrument design is also important because the poorly designed instruments may increase the error associated with localizing points. The intrinsic ability of the tracking hardware to sense and measure the position of instruments plays an obvious role. Each of these factors may be improved and it would be a mistake to assume that current solutions are the optimal ones.

SOFTWARE ENHANCEMENTS

In many operating rooms, rhinologists use the surgical navigation computer as a platform to review preoperative imaging. Interestingly, no system that is commercially available in the United States has a dedicated preoperative planning software option through which a surgeon could review images and plan surgery outside of the operating room. Furthermore, the annotation tools currently available for surgical navigation provide the limited capability of setting a discrete target in ways that are better suited for neurosurgery than otorhinolaryngology. In these systems, active guidance to a specified surgical target is designed for neurosurgical procedures (eg, ventriculostomy), not endoscopic sinus surgery (ESS).

Scopis Building Blocks (Scopis, GmbH, Berlin, Germany) planning software allows the user to annotate a preoperative CT scan to highlight relevant frontal sinus anatomy and the frontal sinus outflow tract (**Fig. 1**).[29,30] The software is based on the so-called building blocks concept, first proposed by Wormald,[31] as a metaphor for conceptualizing complex frontal sinus anatomy. Scopis Building Blocks software is designed so that its preoperative plan can be produced and then imported into the Scopis Hybrid Navigation system. The preoperative plan can be projected as an overlay on the live endoscopic images.[32,33] This system represents an update to the concept of image-enhanced endoscopy, which displayed navigation data as an aligned virtual endoscopic view and real-world endoscopic view in adjacent panels (**Fig. 2**).[34] Both systems require a registration process through which the conventional endoscopic view is aligned with corresponding imaging data.

The development of preoperative planning software is only 1 step. It will be more important to bring that plan into the operating room on the surgical navigation platform. The fusion of the preoperative plan images and the intraoperative views of anatomy will be an important milestone. Ultimately, it is likely that surgical navigation systems will incorporate technology for augmented reality (AR) to combine preoperative imaging data and intraoperative images. In all its forms, AR technology provides an overlay of preoperative imaging on the conventional views of the surgical field.[35,36]

AR may be broadly classified into 2 types. In the first type, the AR projects annotations or other models from the preoperative planning software onto the endoscopic

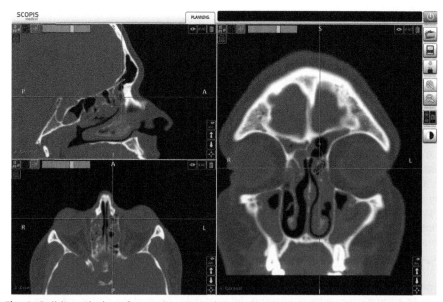

Fig. 1. Building Blocks software (Scopis GmbH, Berlin, Germany) permits the user to annotate the preoperative CT scan. In this instance, the user has marked the ager nasi cell with a green box and the frontal sinus outflow pathway with an orange line. This surgical plan may be imported into the Scopis navigation system. (*Courtesy of* Scopis GmbH, Berlin, Germany; with permission.)

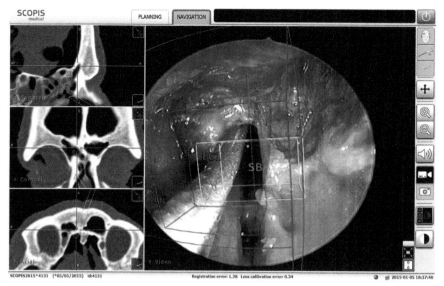

Fig. 2. Scopis Hybrid Navigation (Scopis GmbH, Berlin, Germany) includes AR tools in a cadaveric dissection. In this image, pre-dissection annotations (AN, agger nasi cell; FC1, type 1 frontal cell; SB, suprabullar cell) are projected as an overlay on the endoscopic image and the position of the tracked image tip is shown on the orthogonal CT images. (*Courtesy of* Scopis GmbH, Berlin, Germany; with permission.)

images, as in the Scopis platform previously described. A second alternative it to fuse the real-world endoscopic image to a virtual endoscopy image. This second approach has been tested in a cadaveric laboratory on a prototype system.[37] In both approaches, the surgical navigation system must track the telescope position and register its position relative to the preoperative imaging data set.

Navigation incorporating virtual 3-dimensional (3D) models has also been proposed. Unlike AR (in which the real-world endoscopic images and the virtual data set are merged), virtual 3D navigations systems depict a virtual world typically adjacent to the standard endoscopic images. A randomized, controlled trial of this technology in a cadaveric model did not demonstrate better accuracy with the virtual 3D navigation system.[38] Implicit in AR is that the AR offers meaningful addition (or removal) of visual information on a single image for the user. Obviously, achieving clinically relevant AR will require technical advances as well as considerable efforts for optimizing the user interface and experience.

Intuitively, AR should be an obvious advance over conventional surgical navigation; however, initial experiences suggest that this may not be the case. In a comparison of endoscopy with AR versus conventional endoscopy in a cadaveric simulation of sinus and skull base surgery, users of the AR technology exhibited inattentional blindness (ie, they failed to recognize an unusual finding of skull base violation or foreign body), although users of AR were able to more accurately identify a target.[39] Similar observations have been made in other fields.[40] Thus, the application of AR in the operating room setting will need to mitigate the impact of surgeon's intrinsic perceptual bandwidth limitation. More importantly, AR should provide the most relevant information for the most critical tasks in a user-friendly context.

Dedicated preoperative planning software will also open other advancements for surgical navigation. Safety in ESS often is a task of identifying critical structures (orbit wall, ethmoid roof, optic nerve, internal carotid artery) and avoiding them. If these structures could be tagged or labeled during preoperative planning and those annotations could be visualized during surgery through navigation, this feature may represent yet another enhancement of surgery. In concept, the preoperative planning could involve designating antitargets[32] or no-fly zones, and navigation would provide a proximity warning as a critical structure is approached. A prototype navigation system, which provides visual cues for annotated critical structures, as well as proximity alerts to the same structures during surgical navigation, has been tested in a cadaveric simulation of skull base surgery. Participants had a favorable impression of the technology and the investigators were able to confirm reductions in mental demand, effort, and frustration through the use of the technology.[41,42]

Current navigation systems show preoperative imaging as the standard orthogonal views of axial, coronal, and sagittal slices. In addition, MRIs may be registered to CT images to create hybrid images[43] and CT angiography images may be substituted for noncontrast CT images.[44] Currently, these images may be manipulated but the ability to segment preoperative imaging is quite limited. Specific segmentation protocols, if they were sufficiently automated, may be useful. For instance, the creation of cut views of a 3D of the sinuses may be helpful.

BETTER HARDWARE

The latest generation surgical navigation systems feature a much smaller footprint (**Figs. 3** and **4**). Certainly, this is an important change for the office setting where space is limited in comparison with a standard operating room where this is less of an issue. Even in the operating room, a smaller footprint would permit placement of the surgical navigation system on the same tower as the video equipment. This clearly is more convenient but it also has implications for workflow. A single tower with a single, large dedicated screen creates the opportunity for more efficient delivery of information to the surgeon. If the software is appropriately optimized, navigation may evolve into an active display of endoscopic images and annotated, high-quality preoperative imaging.

Over the years, wireless instrumentation has been offered for surgical navigation. The devices have not been popular because the bulk of the tracking device has always been an issue. In theory advances in miniaturization may permit the development of wireless tools that work well during endoscopic sinus and skull base surgery.

Microsensors for EM tracking systems have been available for many years but only recently have they been incorporated into surgical navigation. Fiagon ENT Navigation and Scopis Hybrid Navigation both feature microsensors tracking (**Fig. 5**). Because microsensors may be placed at the distal end of an instrument, they have a few advantages over trackers placed on the proximal end. A device with a distal microsensor may be made malleable, allowing the surgeon to bend a suction or probe to reach an area that otherwise would be out of reach (**Fig. 6**). A distal microsensor also may make the instrument tracking more reliable because it takes away the impact of bend or flex in the instrument. Finally, microsensors may also be used to guide balloon catheter placement during balloon sinus dilations.[45]

Surgical navigation with balloon catheters may take several different forms. Placing a tracker on the proximal end of an introducer has been proposed,[46] but this approach does not seem to have much clinical utility because it does not really indicate the position of the balloon as it crosses the frontal sinus outflow. Rigid balloon devices with

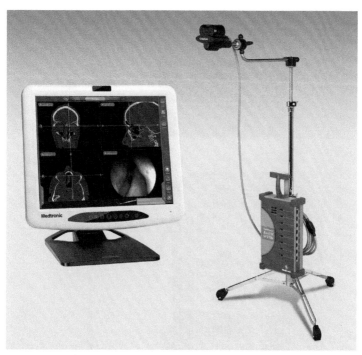

Fig. 3. Fusion Compact (Medtronic, Jacksonville, FL, USA) offers a dramatically reduced footprint. The computer and monitor is a single unit that fits on small table top and the tracking hardware is pole-mounted. This system is ideally suited to an office environment. (*Reprinted* with the permission of Medtronic, Inc. © 2016.)

an EM sensor built into the handle have been available for several years (**Fig. 7**). Flexible or malleable balloon devices will require the use of microsensors. In concept, navigation software may be adjusted to take advantage of the microsensors in balloon catheters. For instance, it would be desirable to lay out the planned trajectory of a balloon catheter during preoperative planning and then track the position of the balloon tip relative to that preoperative planning. Ideally, this approach would include AR-type displays or, at least, screen animations to guide appropriate placement. The impact of microsensors on balloon catheters may be substantial. Although many surgeons report no difficulty with placement of the devices, other experienced surgeons report considerable difficulty.[47] Regardless, the standard technique of transillumination only indicates that the balloon has reached its target but it does not indicate the path to the target. For natural pathway surgery, confirmation of the path to target is important. In addition, transillumination is not an option for the sphenoid sinus and it may be associated with a false positive at the frontal sinus in the presence of specific anatomic configurations (eg, large supraorbital ethmoid sinus or large type 3 frontal cell). Navigation offers the promise of more precise balloon catheter placement.

At least 2 studies have confirmed that intraoperative CT scans demonstrate findings that lead to additional surgical manipulation at 2 academic medical centers with experienced surgeons in approximately 25% of cases.[48,49] Current navigation systems cannot reflect the impact of surgery on the preoperative imaging and this may lead to misconceptions about the completeness of surgery. Unfortunately, intraoperative CT scanners were cumbersome and expensive, and the technology has not been

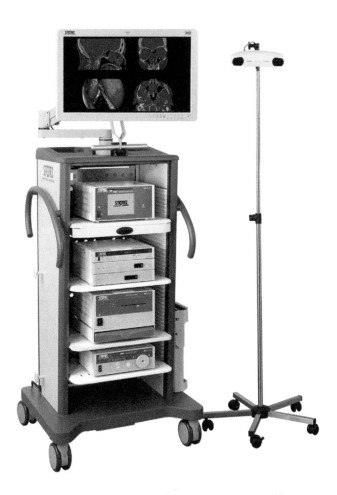

Fig. 4. The optical navigation system from Karl Storz (Tuttlingen, Germany) has a small control box that fits on the endoscopic cart. The camera array is small and may be mounted on a pole. The system shares the same monitor as the endoscopic camera system. (©2016 Photo Courtesy of KARL STORZ Endoscopy-America, Inc.)

widely adapted. Another alternative is to incorporate intraoperative fluoroscopy[50] but this approach is also time-consuming. Nonetheless, there is clearly a role as suggested by the 25% rate of changes triggered by the review of an intraoperative CT scanner. Future navigation systems are likely to incorporate some type of intraoperative update, presumably using portable CT scanners that be easily deployed in the operating room.

For an endoscopic skull base surgery, the need for an intraoperative update is even greater because the violation of the skull base permits the shift of intracranial soft tissues. In theory, a small ultrasound probe that is tracked could provide imaging data that are fused to the preoperative imaging data set. Moreover, an ultrasound would

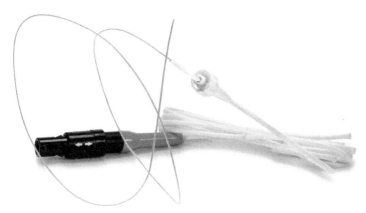

Fig. 5. The Fiagon GuideWire (Fiagon, Berlin, Germany) features a microsensor with outer diameter of 0.5 mm and length of 8 mm. This device may pass through standard devices, including many sinus balloon systems. (*Courtesy of* Fiagon, Berlin, Germany; with permission.)

be ideally suited for confirming the position of a vascular structure, such as the internal carotid artery.

Changes in display technology are likely in future navigation systems. As previously noted, there is certainly a trend for using a larger monitor that displays navigational information and conventional endoscopy images on the same screen. It is interesting to speculate on the possible role of an immersive, head-mounted display (eg, Microsoft HoloLens, Redmond, Washington[51]). This technology does not immerse the viewer in a virtual world; instead, the display projects holograms into real-world images. In concept, technology such as HoloLens, when combined with surgical navigation, may provide the surgeon with a real-time, 3D AR view of the operating field.

GUIDED DRUG DELIVERY

Early in the era of ESS, the goal of sinus surgery was the interruption of the sinusitis cycle through opening blocked sinus ostia. Over the past 15 years, the treatment

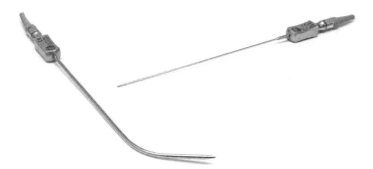

Fig. 6. Tools for the Fiagon navigation platform (Fiagon, Berlin, Germany) include malleable probes. Because the sensor is in the tip of each instrument, each instrument does not need recalibration. The surgeon may bend the instrument as needed. Similar malleable suctions are also available. (*Courtesy of* Fiagon, Berlin, Germany; with permission.)

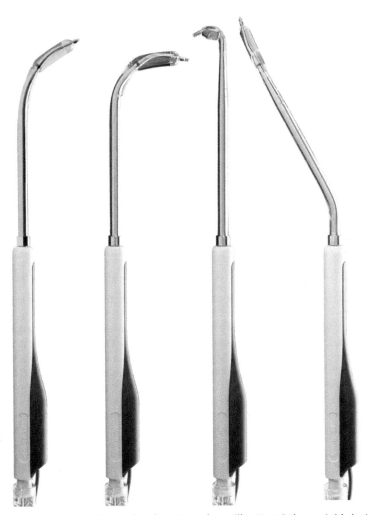

Fig. 7. NuVent balloon catheters (Medtronic, Jacksonville, FL, USA) are rigid devices that include EM sensors, which can be tracked with both the Fusion and Fusion Compact navigation systems. The NuVent family of devices includes 2 frontal sinus balloons, a maxillary balloon, and a sphenoid balloon. (Reprinted with the permission of Medtronic, Inc. © 2016.)

emphasis in the care of patient with of chronic rhinosinusitis has shifted to modulating mucosal inflammation through a combination of sinus surgery (which opens sinuses and thus provides access) and delivery of topical medications (mostly steroids). Thus, budesonide irrigations are widely used, although data from prospective trials are sparse. In addition, some surgeons have adopted the mometasone-releasing steroid implant (PROPEL and PROPEL Mini, Intersect ENT, Menlo Park, CA, USA)[52] as a way to deliver steroids to the surgically opened spaces.[53] In addition, Intersect ENT has released a related product, known as PROPEL Contour, intended for placement after sinus ostial dilatation.[54] Obviously, precise placement of such a device is critical for its therapeutic effect. It is easy to foresee a role for surgical navigation in the placement of PROPEL Contour and future related devices, via natural pathways, with minimal disruptions to sinus anatomy and architecture.

A FUTURE FOR ROBOTICS?

Surgical robots that incorporate surgical navigation have already been developed for both cochlear implantation and mastoidectomy.[55] These robots function in an autonomous or semiautonomous fashion. In contrast, other surgical robots are under the direct control of the surgeon. Within otolaryngology, these robots are used in transoral robotic surgery procedures. Because of the bulk of the available robots, a transantral approach to the skull base has been developed for robotic surgery of the skull base in cadavers.[56] Significant refinements (especially in regard to size and precision) will be necessary for robotic surgery with surgical navigation to become widely accepted in rhinology.

SUMMARY

Surgical navigation has been an important advance for endoscopic sinus and skull base surgery over the past 25 years. By providing localization information relative to preoperative imaging, this technology has facilitated more complex surgery for better patient outcomes. Nonetheless, current surgical navigation systems are not fully optimized. Ideally, the next-generation system will address some (or, it is hoped, all) of these limitations. A critical focus should be on moving surgical navigation error (TRE) closer to 1.0 mm while miminizing the positive skew in the error distribution, a level of accuracy that will stretch technical capabilities but should be feasible. Future systems are also likely to have a smaller footprint and, more importantly, present localization data to the surgeon in novel ways, beyond a simple display of the orthogonal CT scan data. In this regard, AR holds great promise for transforming how surgeons interact with preoperative imaging data at the time of surgery. Of course, specific predictions about technology developments are futile; however, in this instance, it is reasonable to anticipate significant improvements in surgical navigation in response to growing clinical needs and technological advancements.

REFERENCES

1. Hepworth E, Bucknor M, Patel A, et al. Nationwide survey on the use of image-guided functional endoscopic sinus surgery. Otolaryngol Head Neck Surg 2006;135(1):68–73.
2. Orlandi R, Petersen E. Image guidance: a survey of attitudes and use. Am J Rhinol 2006;20(4):406–11.
3. Justice JM, Orlandi RR. An update on attitudes and use of image-guided surgery. Int Forum Allergy Rhinol 2012;2(2):155–9.
4. American Academy of Otolaryngology-Head & Neck Surgery. Position Statement: intra-operative use of computer aided surgery. 2014. Available at: http://www.entnet.org/content/intra-operative-use-computer-aided-surgery. Accessed August 20, 2016.
5. Fried M, Moharir V, Shin J, et al. Comparison of endoscopic sinus surgery with and without image guidance. Am J Rhinol 2002;16:193–7.
6. Metson R, Cosenza M, Gliklich RE, et al. The role of image-guidance systems for head and neck surgery. Arch Otolaryngol Head Neck Surg 1999;125: 1100–4.
7. Javer AR, Genoway KA. Patient quality of life improvements with and without computer assistance in sinus surgery: outcomes study. J Otolaryngol 2006; 35(6):373–9.

8. Masterson L, Agalato E, Pearson C. Image-guided sinus surgery: practical and financial experiences from a UK centre 2001-2009. J Laryngol Otol 2012; 126(12):1224–30.

9. Tabaee A, Kassenoff T, Kacker A, et al. The efficacy of computer assisted surgery in the endoscopic management of cerebrospinal fluid rhinorrhea. Otolaryngol Head Neck Surg 2005;133(6):936–43.

10. Tabaee A, Hsu A, Shrime M, et al. Quality of life and complications following image-guided endoscopic sinus surgery. Otolaryngol Head Neck Surg 2006; 135(1):76–80.

11. Dubin MR, Tabaee A, Scrugges JT, et al. Image-guided endoscopic orbital decompression for Graves' orbitopathy. Ann Otol Rhinol Laryngol 2008;117(3):177–85.

12. Tscopp KP, Thomaser EG. Outcome of functional endonasal sinus surgery with and without CT-navigation. Rhinology 2008;46:116–20.

13. Reardon E. Navigation risks associated with sinus surgery and clinical effects of implementing a navigational system for sinus surgery. Laryngoscope 2002;112:1–19.

14. Rombaux P, Ledeghen S, Hamoir M, et al. Computer-assisted surgery and endoscopic endonasal approach in 32 procedures. Acta Otorhinolaryngol Belg 2003; 57:131–7.

15. Eliashar R, Sichel J-Y, Gross M, et al. Image-guided navigation system–a new technology for complex endoscopic endonasal surgery. Postgrad Med J 2003; 79:686–90.

16. Al-Swiahb JN, Al Dousary SH. Computer-aided endoscopic sinus surgery: a retrospective comparative study. Ann Saudi Med 2010;30(2):149–52.

17. Strauss G, Koulechov K, Rottger S, et al. Evaluation of a navigation system for ENT with surgical efficiency criteria. Laryngoscope 2006;116(4):564–72.

18. Mueller SA, Caversaccio M. Outcome of computer-assisted surgery in patients with chronic rhinosinusitis. J Laryngol Otol 2010;124(5):500–4.

19. Ramakrishnan V, Orlandi R, Citardi M, et al. The use of image-guided surgery in endoscopic sinus surgery: an evidence-based review with recommendations. Int Forum Allergy Rhinol 2013;3(3):236–41.

20. Smith T, Stewart M, Orlandi R, et al. Indications for image-guided sinus surgery: The current evidence. Am J Rhinol 2007;21(1):80–3.

21. Dalgorf DM, Sacks R, Wormald PJ, et al. Image-guided surgery influences perioperative morbidity from endoscopic sinus surgery: a systematic review and meta-analysis. Otolaryngol Head Neck Surg 2013;149(1):17–29.

22. Chang CM, Jaw FS, Lo WC, et al. Three-dimensional analysis of the accuracy of optic and electromagnetic navigation systems using surface registration in live endoscopic sinus surgery. Rhinology 2016;54(1):88–94.

23. Knott PD, Batra PS, Citardi MJ. Computer aided surgery: concepts and applications in rhinology. Otolaryngol Clin North Am 2006;39(3):503–22, ix.

24. Labadie RF, Davis BM, Fitzpatrick JM. Image-guided surgery: what is the accuracy? Curr Opin Otolaryngol Head Neck Surg 2005;13:27–31.

25. Olson G, Citardi M. Image-guided functional endoscopic sinus surgery. Otolaryngol Head Neck Surg 2000;123(3):188–94.

26. Stryker. Pattern Recognition Optics for Functional Endoscopic Sinus Surgery. Available at: http://www.stryker.com/en-us/products/OREquipmentConnectivity/ SurgicalNavigation/SurgicalNavigationSoftware/PROFESSNavigationSystem/ index.htm. Accessed August 20, 2016.

27. Fiagon. ENT navigation: safer, faster and simpler with Fiagon. Available at: http:// www.fiagon.com/tracey/. Accessed March 9, 2017.

28. KARL STORZ GmbH & Co. KG. Available at: https://www.karlstorz.com/ee/en/highlights-nav.htm?d=HM&s=NAV#mod-9718. Accessed March 8, 2017.

29. Scopis Medical. Experience the Advanced 3D Sinus Surgery Planning with Scopis Building Blocks planning software. Available at: http://planning.scopis.com/. Accessed March 9, 2017.

30. Agbetoba A, Luong A, Siow JK, et al. Educational Utility of advanced 3-dimensional virtual imaging in evaluating the anatomical configuration of the frontal recess. Int Forum Allergy Rhinol 2016;7:143–8.

31. Wormald P-J. Three-dimensional building block approach to understanding the anatomy of the frontal recess and frontal sinus. Oper Tech Otolayngol Head Neck Surg 2006;17(1):2–5.

32. Citardi MJ, Agbetoba A, Bigcas JL, et al. Augmented reality for endoscopic sinus surgery with surgical navigation: a cadaver study. Int Forum Allergy Rhinol 2016;6(5):523–8.

33. Winne C, Khan M, Stopp F, et al. Overlay visualization in endoscopic ENT surgery. Int J Comput Assist Radiol Surg 2011;6(3):401–6.

34. Shahidi R, Bax MR, Maurer CR Jr, et al. Implementation, calibration and accuracy testing of an image-enhanced endoscopy system. IEEE Trans Med Imaging 2002;21(12):1524–35.

35. Besharati Tabrizi L, Mahvash M. Augmented reality-guided neurosurgery: accuracy and intraoperative application of an image projection technique. J Neurosurg 2015;123(1):206–11.

36. Suzuki N, Hattori A, Limura J, et al. Development of AR surgical navigation systems for multiple regions. Stud Health Technol Inform 2014;196:404–8.

37. Li L, Yang J, Chu Y, et al. A novel augmented reality navigation system for endoscopic sinus and skull base surgery: a feasibility study. PLoS One 2016;11(1):e0146996.

38. Dixon BJ, Chan H, Daly MJ, et al. Three-dimensional virtual navigation versus conventional image guidance: A randomized controlled trial. Laryngoscope 2016;126(7):1510–5.

39. Dixon BJ, Daly MJ, Chan HH, et al. Inattentional blindness increased with augmented reality surgical navigation. Am J Rhinol Allergy 2014;28(5):433–7.

40. Yeh MM. Display signaling in augmented reality: effects of cue reliability and image realism on attention allocation and trust calibration. Hum Factors 2001;43(3):355–65.

41. Dixon BJ, Daly MJ, Chan H, et al. Augmented real-time navigation with critical structure proximity alerts for endoscopic skull base surgery. Laryngoscope 2014;124(4):853–9.

42. Dixon BJ, Chan H, Daly MJ, et al. The effect of augmented real-time image guidance on task workload during endoscopic sinus surgery. Int Forum Allergy Rhinol 2012;2(5):405–10.

43. Leong JL, Batra PS, Citardi MJ. CT-MR image fusion for the management of skull base lesions. Otolaryngol Head Neck Surg 2006;134(5):868–76.

44. Leong JL, Batra PS, Citardi MJ. Three-dimensional computed tomography angiography of the internal carotid artery for preoperative evaluation of sinonasal lesions and intraoperative surgical navigation. Laryngoscope 2005;115(9):1618–23.

45. Lam K BJ, Luong A, Yao W, et al. Balloon sinus ostial dilatation with microsensor navigation in the operating room setting. 2015.

46. Leventhal D, Heffelfinger R, Rosen M. Using image guidance tracking during balloon catheter dilation of sinus ostia. Otolaryngol Head Neck Surg 2007;137: 341–2.

47. Tomazic PV, Stammberger H, Braun H, et al. Feasibility of balloon sinuplasty in patients with chronic rhinosinusitis: the Graz experience. Rhinology 2013;51(2): 120–7.

48. Batra PS, Kanowitz SJ, Citardi MJ. Clinical utility of intraoperative volume computed tomography scanner for endoscopic sinonasal and skull base procedures. Am J Rhinol 2008;22(5):511–5.

49. Jackman AH, Palmer JN, Chiu AG, et al. Use of intraoperative CT scanning in endoscopic sinus surgery: a preliminary report. Am J Rhinol 2008;22(2):170–4.

50. Brown S, Sadoughi B, Cuellar H, et al. Feasibility of near real-time image-guided sinus surgery using intraoperative fluoroscopic computed axial tomography. Otolaryngol Head Neck Surg 2007;136(2):268–73.

51. Microsoft. HoloLens. Available at: https://www.microsoft.com/microsoft-hololens/en-us. Accessed August 21, 2016.

52. Marple BF, Smith TL, Han JK, et al. Advance II: a prospective, randomized study assessing safety and efficacy of bioabsorbable steroid-releasing sinus implants. Otolaryngol Head Neck Surg 2012;146(6):1004–11.

53. Kennedy DW. The PROPEL[trademark] steroid-releasing bioabsorbable implant to improve outcomes of sinus surgery. Expert Rev Respir Med 2012;6:493.

54. Intersect ENT. Available at: http://www.intersectent.com/wp-content/uploads/Contour-FDA-FINAL.pdf. Accessed March 8, 2017.

55. Dillon NP. A compact, bone-attached robot for mastoidectomy. J Med Device 2015;9(3):0310031–7.

56. Hanna EY. Robotic endoscopic surgery of the skull base: a novel surgical approach. Arch Otolaryngol Head Neck Surg 2007;133(12):1209–14.

Robotics in Sinus and Skull Base Surgery

Sanjeet Rangarajan, MD, MEng[a], Ralph Abi Hachem, MD[b], Enver Ozer, MD[c],
Andre Beer-Furlan, MD[d], Daniel Prevedello, MD[e], Ricardo L. Carrau, MD[c,*]

KEYWORDS

- Robotic surgery • Sinonasal • Skull base • Sinus surgery

KEY POINTS

- Robots have been present in medicine for more than 30 years; however, recent advances have introduced many advantages, including high definition, 3-dimensional visualization, tremor-free surgery, and the ability to translate macro-movements into fine, precise maneuvers.
- The Food and Drug Administration has approved two robotic surgery systems for use in the head and neck: the da Vinci Surgical System (Intuitive Surgical, Inc, Sunnyvale, CA) and the Medrobotics Flex Robotic System (Medrobotics Corp, Raynham, MA). Several approaches and techniques have been described in the literature, demonstrating that both systems are capable of accessing the sinonasal cavity and cranial base.
- Several technical challenges remain before widespread use of robotic systems within the sinonasal corridor will be possible, including lack of haptic feedback, absence of drills and bone cutting instruments, and the large size of the instruments.

INTRODUCTION

Since the 1980s, when a robot was first used to assist surgeons performing an intracranial biopsy,[1] modern robotic-assisted surgery (RAS) has burgeoned into a versatile tool for surgical teams practicing in a variety of specialties, including urology,

Disclosures: None.
[a] Department of Otolaryngology–Head and Neck Surgery, The Ohio State University Wexner Medical Center, Columbus, OH 43210, USA; [b] Division of Head and Neck Surgery & Communication Sciences, Department of Surgery, Duke University Medical Center, Durham, NC 27710, USA; [c] Department of Otolaryngology–Head and Neck Surgery, The Ohio State University Wexner Medical Center, Starling Loving Hall, Room B221, 320 West 10th Avenue, Columbus, OH 43210, USA; [d] Department of Neurological Surgery, The Ohio State University Wexner Medical Center, Columbus, OH 43210, USA; [e] Department of Neurological Surgery, The Ohio State University Wexner Medical Center, Doan Hall 410 West 10th Avenue, Room N1011-A, Columbus, OH 43210, USA
* Corresponding author. Department of Otolaryngology–Head & Neck Surgery, The Ohio State University Wexner Medical Center, Starling Loving Hall, Room B221, 320 West 10th Avenue, Columbus, OH 43210.
E-mail address: Ricardo.Carrau@osumc.edu

Otolaryngol Clin N Am 50 (2017) 633–641
http://dx.doi.org/10.1016/j.otc.2017.01.013
0030-6665/17/© 2017 Elsevier Inc. All rights reserved.
oto.theclinics.com

gynecology, abdominal surgery, neurosurgery, and cardiothoracic surgery. When considering the overall history of robots in medicine, the use of these tools in otolaryngology has emerged relatively recently.

Transoral robotic surgery (TORS) has been proven to be safe and to yield acceptable oncological and functional outcomes for surgery of the oropharynx, hypopharynx, supraglottis, and glottis. TORS has been successful at reducing morbidity, improving quality of life, and providing access to areas that previously required mandibulotomy or other more radical approaches in the past. TORS has changed the paradigm of management of tumors in these anatomic locations.

Compared with TORS, robotic-assisted approaches to the sinonasal corridor and skull base are still at an early stage of development; but some success has been reported over the past few years. Some of these systems offer immersive, high-resolution visualization and the ability to translate human macro-movements into fine, precise robotic manipulation of tissue, which are prized commodities in sinonasal and endoscopic skull base surgery. In this article, the authors review the recent literature discussing the role of robotic surgery in managing sinonasal and skull base pathologic conditions and discuss its current advantages and limitations.

AVAILABLE ROBOTIC SYSTEMS AND INSTRUMENTATION

The terms *robot*, *robotic assisted*, and *robotic surgery* have been applied loosely to many different tools and systems over the years. As mentioned earlier, the first reported robotic-assisted surgical procedure was reported in 1985 by Kwoh and colleagues,[1] who used a PUMA 560 industrial robot originally developed for General Motors to stereotactically guide surgeons performing an intracranial biopsy of a suspicious brain lesion. Although the robot indeed pointed toward the desired target, the physical biopsy was still performed by the surgeons' hands in the traditional manner.

Over the last 30 years, advances have led to a series of devices that allow for either visualization (eg, the SOLOASSIST automated endoscope holder[2]) or instrumentation (eg, the Vanderbilt concentric tube continuum robot) within the sinonasal cavity/anterior skull base; however, systems that can perform both functions and truly be called robotic surgery systems are few.

Currently, there are only 2 Food and Drug Administration (FDA)–approved surgical robotic systems that allow both visualization and instrumentation and have been used to access the sinonasal cavity and skull base in cadaveric, animal, and human subjects: the da Vinci Surgical System (Intuitive Surgical, Inc, Sunnyvale, CA) and the Medrobotics Flex Robotic System (Medrobotics Corp, Raynham, MA). The authors describe each in this section.

- The Medrobotics Flex Robotic System is the newest robotic surgery system and was approved for use in the United States in July 2015. It was specifically designed for use in the oropharynx, hypopharynx, and larynx. The primary advantage of the Flex system lies in the maneuverability of its endoscope and accompanying instrumentation, offering a flexible endoscopic system capable of steering around obstructing anatomy with 102° of freedom. The system consists of a main console that houses a touchscreen monitor and physician control joystick as well as a base unit that contains the endoscope and instrumentation components. The system contains 2 working channels that can accommodate a wide variety of instruments. In spite of its flexible, steerable configuration, the large diameter of the endoscope and instrumentation preclude a purely endonasal approach to the skull base. Schuler and colleagues[3] demonstrated a successful endoscopic visualization of the anterior skull base using the Flex system;

however, midfacial degloving was required to accommodate the robotic arms. In their study, the Flex endoscope was used for visualization, whereas the actual surgical maneuvers were performed using standard, conventional instrumentation. The robotic arms were able to reach pertinent anatomic landmarks, but they did not perform any actual procedural tasks. The Flex system also does not provide haptic feedback or stereotactic navigation, both desired features in endoscopic sinonasal and skull base surgery.

- The da Vinci Surgical System is the most widely used robotic surgical system in the United States; its applications have been well documented in the otolaryngology literature, although it was not initially designed with the head and neck in mind. The da Vinci system consists of several different components working in concert: A main console that serves as the control center where the surgeon is seated, a patient-side surgical robot equipped with a 3-dimensional (3D) rigid endoscope, and a video display cart. The endoscopes for use in the newest version of the system (Xi) are 8.5 mm in diameter and have 0° and 30° viewing angles available. The entire endoscope arm can pivot, rotate, and translate to change the operator's view; however, it is rigid and cannot bend or change its trajectory significantly once within the surgical field. The endoscope, which is fit with a dual-lens, 3-CCD (Charge-coupled device) camera, gives the operating surgeon a high-definition, stereoscopic view of the surgical field. Various instrument attachments as small as 5 mm in diameter can be introduced into one of 2 to 3 robotic arms and are designed to operate with 7° of freedom based on the wristed movements of the operating surgeon.

The da Vinci system has been used in head and neck surgery since 2005[4] and has the benefit of having already been through several product cycles since its initial launch. The relative maturity of the da Vinci product line when compared with the only other surgical robot system cleared for use in the United States affords certain feature advantages. The newest version of the da Vinci Surgical System is the da Vinci Xi, which offers several improvements over its predecessors.[5] One of these is the automatic configuration of its boom arms based on endoscopic and laser guidance, a feature that reduces the setup time, which has been a common source of criticism.[6] Nonetheless, even this current iteration does not provide the surgeon with haptic feedback or stereotactic navigation features.

Neither system has been demonstrated to have the ability to access the sinonasal cavity or anterior skull base using a purely endonasal approach, instead requiring additional morbidity through traditional open approaches that have been used more selectively over the last 15 years as expanded endonasal approaches have gained favor. A common limiting factor of both systems is the size of their endoscopes and instrumentation. The typical rigid endoscope used during endonasal skull base surgery is only 4 mm in diameter, and each instrument manually inserted in the nose during a typical approach is only on the order of millimeters. To create steerable robotic instrumentation capable of navigating the sinonasal cavity, a team at Vanderbilt has developed a prototype system using concentric tube robotic arms, allowing tentacle-like motion and manipulation.[7] In addition to these systems, there are several automated endoscope holders and positioning systems, which allow for hands-free visualization but do not have instrument arms to truly be considered fully robotic solutions.[2]

Further limitations of both FDA approved systems are the lack of a high-speed drill, which is required to remove the hard bone of the sinonasal cavity and skull base and the lack of adequate suctioning capacity. In addition, the lack of haptic feedback is a significant barrier to practical use in sinonasal and skull base surgery. Haptic feedback is an extremely active area of study within robotics and of utmost importance in dissection within anatomically sensitive areas, such as the skull base. Alternatives to overcome these hurdles are being actively investigated across the world. A feasibility study was recently performed by a team at the University of Pennsylvania to investigate haptic feedback in transoral robotic surgery, a concept that may transfer to endonasal surgery in the near future.[8]

SURGICAL ROUTES TO THE SINONASAL CAVITIES AND SKULL BASE

Given that instruments developed for the two previously developed FDA-approved robotic surgery systems are not ergonomically designed to fit the sinonasal cavities, additional improvisations and surgical routes have been described that optimize access to the cranial base. These approaches have been mostly performed within the context of cadaveric studies and have been minimally used for live patients.

Combined Transnasal and Transantral Approach

In 2007, Hanna and colleagues[9] described a surgical approach to the cranial fossa using the da Vinci robot on 4 frozen cadavers via a combined transnasal-transantral approach.

Technique
Access to the sinonasal cavities is gained through bilateral superior vestibular/sublabial incisions followed by a wide anterior and middle maxillary antrostomy (similar to a Caldwell-Luc). A posterior septectomy is performed joining both sinonasal cavities into one surgical field. Then the da Vinci robot is docked at the head of the bed; the camera arm port is introduced through the nostril and the right and left robotic arm ports through the respective anterior and middle antrostomies into the nasal cavity. Then a total ethmoidectomy, wide common sphenoidotomy, and resection of the middle and superior turbinates are performed using the robot, providing access to the anterior and middle cranial fossa. The cribriform plate is resected, and the dural defect is then sutured closed using a graft in a watertight fashion with 6 to 0 nylon sutures. This approach provides excellent access to the anterior and central skull base. The investigators emphasized the ability to perform 2-handed tremor-free suture and closure of dural defects.[9,10] The use of traditional surgical drills was not described. Cho and colleagues[11] described a similar combined endonasal-transantral approach for robotic nasopharyngectomy.

Combined Transnasal and Transcervical Approach

The combined transnasal and transcervical approach was developed by Dallan and colleagues[12] to avoid damage to the teeth in dentate patients using a transoral port.

Technique
Similar to the cervical-TORS (C-TORS), it involves the placement of transcervical paramandibular trocars by performing a small cervical incision at the angle of the mandible, then reaching the oral cavity through blunt subperiosteal dissection. The trocars are directed through the oropharynx superiorly into the nasopharynx. Then a posterior septectomy is performed to improve visualization of the operative field, reduce conflict between the instruments, and increase maneuverability. The skull base is removed using a conventional endonasal technique with drills and rongeurs, and then the da Vinci robot is used to dissect the posterior cranial fossa and pituitary region. This approach

provides a superior access to the sella, suprasellar region, clivus, optic chiasm, and pons with the ability to perform a robotic pituitary transposition.

Combined Expanded Endonasal Approach and Transoral Approach (Extended Endonasal Approach–Transoral Robotic Surgery)

This approach was described by Carrau and colleagues[13] in 2013, practiced on cadavers, and then applied to 2 patients. The extended endonasal approach (EEA)-TORS technique was used on human subjects to (1) resect an adenoid cystic carcinoma of the nasopharynx with extension both laterally into the infratemporal fossa and inferiorly below the level of the hard palate and (2) resect a clival chordoma with extension into the craniocervical junction inferiorly to C2. Both patients had gross total resection with no complications and minimal postoperative morbidity.

Technique

The first step of the dissection is to provide a sinonasal corridor using an endoscopic endonasal technique. It includes ipsilateral resection of the inferoposterior half of the middle turbinate, maxillary antrostomy, total ethmoidectomy, and a wide sphenoidotomy. The next step is a Denker approach, which entails removal of the pyriform aperture, anterior maxillary wall, inferior turbinate, and lateral nasal wall, thus, providing full access to the posterior and lateral maxillary wall. A posterior septectomy is done to optimize binostril access. The sphenoid floor is drilled to be flush with the clivus. The vidian nerve and maxillary nerve (V2) are followed proximally to identify the junction of the paraclival and petrous carotid artery. The pterygoid process is drilled exposing the eustachian tube, mandibular nerve (V3), and middle cranial fossa. The pterygoid and tensor veli palatine muscles are resected or mobilized exposing the parapharyngeal internal carotid artery (ICA), which constitutes the danger zone and lateral limit of dissection in endoscopic nasopharyngectomy. Once the inferior-most limit using EEA was reached at the level of the eustachian tube, the da Vinci robot is brought into position. A Crowe-Davis mouth gag is inserted. The soft palate is retracted using a red rubber catheter inserted into the nose and pulled through the mouth. A Maryland dissector, a spatula-tip monopolar cautery, and a 0° robotic arm are inserted into the mouth. The superior aspect of the palatoglossal arch is incised, and the inferomedial border of the medial pterygoid muscle is dissected identifying the parapharyngeal fat and ICA. The styloid process and musculature are identified. Further dissection lateral to the parapharyngeal ICA exposes cranial nerves IX to XII and the internal jugular vein. The pterygoid muscles are transected at their mandibular insertion. Then the dissection is extended medially connecting it with the inferior border of the EEA dissection and completion of the nasopharyngectomy with resection of the eustachian tube.

The EEA-TORS approach provides excellent exposure to the posterior skull base, nasopharynx, and infratemporal fossa. The main benefits of combining TORS to EEA to manage skull base tumors is the ability to reach the posterior skull base below the level of the eustachian tube, which is the inferior limit of the EEA, and subsequently achieve a complete resection of the tumor's inferior margin with potential en bloc resection.

Purely Transoral Approach

As the first documented uses of robots in head and neck surgery were for transoral resections of oropharyngeal cancers, a transoral route to the skull base was a natural extension for the University of Pennsylvania group who described this approach in 2007.[14] This approach was aimed at dissecting the parapharyngeal and infratemporal space and was initially tested on cadavers and then subsequently on a live dog. It was then applied to a patient with a benign cystic lesion of the parapharyngeal and infratemporal space.

Technique

The da Vinci robot is docked at the head of the bed. A Crowe-Davis mouth gag retractor (Storz, Heidelberg, Germany) is used to open the oral cavity and expose the oropharynx. The camera and both robotic arms are introduced transorally. The procedure starts with incisions lateral to the anterior tonsillar pillar, followed by dissection of the branches of the external carotid, the jugular vein, internal carotid, and cranial nerves IX, X, XI, and XII. The styloid and pterygoid musculatures are subsequently released to gain lateral access within the infratemporal fossa. Although this proved the feasibility of robotic surgery of the parapharyngeal space and infratemporal fossa, there were major limitations noted and reproduced throughout other experimental studies. The main limitations noted were the lack of drills and rongeurs to remove the skull base bone and the inability of wide resection, thus, precluding its use for malignant lesions. The transoral approach was also described to access the craniocervical junction; however, drilling of the odontoid and arch of C1 was done by an assistant using a conventional technique.[15]

Combined Transcervical and Transoral Approach (Cervical–Transoral Robotic Surgery)

O'Malley and Weinstein[16] described the C-TORS of the skull base on one cadaver.

Technique

The approach entails placement of a 30° high-magnification angled endoscope camera transorally and the effector robotic arms transcervically. The da Vinci robotic arms are introduced via bilateral incision along the posterior margin of both submandibular glands with blind blunt placement of trocars directed superomedially into the oral cavity and accessing the ventral skull base and nasopharynx through the oropharynx. This technique enables surgical dissection in the sphenoid sinus, clivus, sella, and suprasellar fossa with improved instrument angulation and access.

Combined Transnasal and Transoral Approach (CTTP)

A combined transnasal and transoral approach was described by Dallan and colleagues[12] in 2012 and Ozer and colleagues[17] in 2013.

Technique

The setting includes the da Vinci robot docked cranially at the head of the cadaver with a 30° upward-facing lens placed transnasally, a Maryland dissector (Intuitive Surgical, Inc, Sunnyvale, CA), and a cauterization device with a spatula tip placed transorally and used for dissection. The dissection starts with a midline incision in the posterior nasopharyngeal wall followed by bilateral medial to lateral heminasopharyngectomy including resection of the Eustachian tube. This technique provides an optimal approach to the nasopharynx and posterior skull base, especially in edentulous patients given the transoral access without the need to split the palate. Furthermore, the dissection work is done under typical endonasal endoscopic vision, thus, providing the surgeon a more familiar anatomy compared with the purely transoral technique, whereby dissection occurs in down-to-up fashion. This approach can be augmented by going through the hard palate (transpalatal) after elevation of a posteriorly based U-shaped palatal flap and removing the hard palate bone.[17]

Combined Transoral and Midline Suprahyoid Approach

McCool and colleagues[18] described a cadaveric dissection using a midline suprahyoid approach to the infratemporal fossa with the da Vinci robot.

Technique

The approach entails a midline 15-mm incision at the level of the hyoid bone with blunt dissection to gain access into the vallecula. The midline port is placed through the suprahyoid incision. Then a 30° camera is placed transorally in the midline, and the second robotic arm is placed transorally contralateral to the site of dissection. An incision is made in the posterior tonsillar pillar and carried superiorly along the salpingopharyngeal fold. The superior pharyngeal constrictor and the medial pterygoid muscle are divided identifying the lingual and inferior alveolar nerve. Then the internal and external carotid arteries are identified posterior and medial to cranial nerve V3. The middle meningeal artery is dissected up to foramen spinosum. The dissection is extended posteriorly to the jugular foramen identifying the internal jugular vein and cranial nerves IX to XII. The da Vinci robot was used to place surgical clips using an 8-mm clip applier. The combined transoral suprahyoid approach provides a central port access with a low risk of damaging neurovascular structures, thus, allowing dissection of the central and lateral skull base.

Transoral Approach to the Nasopharynx

Robotic surgery of the nasopharynx was initially described in a cadaveric model in 2008 by Ozer and Waltonen[19] followed by subsequent case reports of robotic or robotic-assisted nasopharyngectomy. Tsang and colleagues[20] published a case series of 12 patients who underwent TORS/TORS-assisted nasopharyngectomy. The ideal indication for a robotic nasopharyngectomy is small recurrent nasopharyngeal carcinoma involving the roof or posterior wall of the nasopharynx or the fossa of Rosenmüller, without intranasal or pterygopalatine fossa extension and more than 1 cm away from the ICA. The course of the ICA should not be medial to the medial pterygoid plate. In this approach, tumors abutting or invading the floor of the sphenoid sinus require an additional endoscopic endonasal approach to achieve gross total resection with negative margins. Contraindications to a pure robotic nasopharyngectomy include tumors extending into the pterygopalatine and infratemporal fossa, or less than 1 cm from the ICA, or with retropharyngeal lymph node metastasis or maxillary sinus invasion.

Technique

Patients are positioned in Trendelenburg with the head slightly extended and are orally intubated using a nonkinking endotracheal tube placed over the central lower lip. A Dingman mouth gag retractor is used to expose the palate and oropharynx. The soft palate is divided under direct visualization and retracted laterally. The da Vinci robot is docked at the head of the bed, and a 0° or 30° 8-mm dual channel camera is introduced transorally. Then, using the 5-mm Maryland grasping forceps mounted to the left robotic arm and a monopolar diathermy mounted to the right robotic arm, the nasopharyngeal soft tissue is dissected in an inferior to superior direction and laterally between the carotid arteries. The medial crus of the torus tubarius can be included in the specimen if needed. The dissection is carried through the soft tissue down to the clival bone. Peripheral margins are checked intraoperatively with a frozen section. The defect can be covered using a free mucosal graft or a nasoseptal flap if the carotid is exposed.[20,21]

SUMMARY

Currently, robotic surgery within the sinonasal cavity and skull base is still in its infancy. There is significant promise for purely robotic surgery and RAS to treat sinonasal and skull base pathologies; current devices do have several advantages over traditional methods, including 3D visualization and tremor-free surgery with ability to translate large macro-movements into fine precise tissue manipulations. These features are extremely attractive for surgeons who are used to working in an extremely confined space like the sinonasal cavity. The lack of haptic feedback, the lack of availability of drills and bone cutting instrumentation, and the overall bulkiness of the endoscope and instrument arms pose significant barriers when evaluating the current technology's application to the sinonasal cavity. Previous advances in endoscopic endonasal approaches have allowed our field to treat a multitude of pathologies in an expanding number of locations within the paranasal sinuses and skull base while minimizing patient morbidity. As the authors' review of the literature has demonstrated, existing robotic surgery systems have been adapted to use in the cranial base only by using multiple approaches, not simply the endonasal corridor. The advanced technical skills required and lack of larger human subject series are still major drawbacks to these approaches and together with current technological limitations serve as the main barriers to the widespread utility of robotic sinonasal and skull base surgery.

REFERENCES

1. Kwoh YS, Hou J, Jonckheere EA, et al. A robot with improved absolute positioning accuracy for CT guided stereotactic brain surgery. IEEE Trans Biomed Eng 1988;35:153–61.
2. Kristin J, Geiger R, Kraus P, et al. Assessment of the endoscopic range of motion for head and neck surgery using the SOLOASSIST endoscope holder. Int J Med Robot 2015;11(4):418–23.
3. Schuler PJ, Scheithauer M, Rotter N, et al. A single-port operator-controlled flexible endoscope system for endoscopic skull base surgery. HNO 2015;63(3):189–94.
4. McLeod KI, Melder PC. Da Vinci robot-assisted excision of a vallecular cyst: a case report. Ear Nose Throat J 2005;84(3):170–2.
5. Available at: http://www.intuitivesurgical.com/products/da-vinci-xi/. daVinci Xi Surgical System.
6. Gettman M. Innovations in robotic surgery. Curr Opin Urol 2016;26(3):271–6.
7. Swaney PJ, Gilbert HB, Webster RJ 3rd, et al. Endonasal skull base tumor removal using concentric tube continuum robots: a phantom study. J Neurol Surg B Skull Base 2015 Mar;76(2):145.
8. Bur AM, Gomez ED, Newman JG, et al. Haptic feedback in transoral robotic surgery: a feasibility study. Annual Meeting of the Triologic Society at the Combined Otolaryngology Spring Meetings. 2015.
9. Hanna EY, Holsinger C, DeMonte F, et al. Robotic endoscopic surgery of the skull base. A novel surgical approach. Arch Otolaryngol Head Neck Surg 2007;133:1209–14.
10. Kupferman ME, Demonte F, Levine N, et al. Feasibility of a robotic surgical approach to reconstruct the skull base. Skull Base 2011;21(2):79–82.
11. Cho HJ, Kang JW, Min HJ, et al. Robotic nasopharyngectomy via combined endonasal and transantral port: a preliminary cadaveric study. Laryngoscope 2015;125(8):1839–43.

12. Dallan I, Castelnuovo P, Seccia V, et al. Combined transnasal transcervical robotic dissection of posterior skull base: feasibility in a cadaveric model. Rhinology 2012;50(2):165–70.
13. Carrau RL, Prevedello DM, de Lara D, et al. Combined transoral robotic surgery and endoscopic endonasal approach for the resection of extensive malignancies of the skull base. Head Neck 2013;35(11):E351–8.
14. O'Malley BW Jr, Weinstein GS. Robotic skull base surgery: preclinical investigations to human clinical application. Arch Otolaryngol Head Neck Surg 2007; 133(12):1215–9.
15. Lee JY, O'Malley BW, Newman JG, et al. Transoral robotic surgery of craniocervical junction and atlantoaxial spine: a cadaveric study. J Neurosurg Spine 2010;12:13–8.
16. O'Malley BW Jr, Weinstein GS. Robotic anterior and midline skull base surgery: preclinical investigations. Int J Radiat Oncol Biol Phys 2007;69(2 Suppl):S125–8.
17. Ozer E, Durmus K, Carrau RL, et al. Applications of transoral, transcervical, transnasal, and transpalatal corridors for robotic surgery of the skull base. Laryngoscope 2013;123(9):2176–9.
18. McCool RR, Warren FM, Wiggins RH, et al. Robotic surgery of the infratemporal fossa utilizing novel suprahyoid port. Laryngoscope 2010;120:1738–43.
19. Ozer E, Waltonen J. Transoral robotic nasopharyngectomy: a novel approach for nasopharyngeal lesions. Laryngoscope 2008;118:1613–6.
20. Tsang RK, To VS, Ho AC, et al. Early results of robotic assisted nasopharyngectomy for recurrent nasopharyngeal carcinoma. Head Neck 2015;37(6):788–93.
21. Wei WI, Ho WK. Transoral robotic resection of recurrent nasopharyngeal carcinoma. Laryngoscope 2010;120(10):2011–4.

Endoscopic Skull Base Reconstruction
An Evolution of Materials and Methods

Aaron C. Sigler, DO, MS[a], Brian D'Anza, MD[b],
Brian C. Lobo, MD[c], Troy D. Woodard, MD[d],
Pablo F. Recinos, MD[e], Raj Sindwani, MD, FACS[d],*

KEYWORDS

- Nasoseptal flap • CSF leak repair • Skull base defect repair • Pericranial flap
- Endoscopic endonasal approach • Graduated approach to reconstruction

KEY POINTS

- Certain independent factors affect the decision-making process in selecting the appropriate repair type and the use of a vascularized flap, including size/extent of skull base defect, entrance into an intracranial cistern or ventricle, disorder type (eg, craniopharyngioma, meningioma), disease process (Cushing disease), and body habitus (morbid obesity).
- Cerebrospinal fluid (CSF) leak type (divided among no leak, low flow, and high flow) is a major factor guiding selection of the appropriate repair type.
- Repair of endoscopic skull base defects and CSF leaks in general can include synthetic and autologous dural replacement grafts, free autografts, local and distal vascularized flaps, and even free tissue transfer.
- A graduated laddered approach to skull base reconstruction provides a framework to guide selection of repair technique to ensure a successful outcome while minimizing morbidity for the patient.

[a] Tulane Center for Clinical Neurosciences, Department of Neurosurgery, 131 S. Robertson St., Ste 1300, New Orleans, LA 70112, USA; [b] Section of Rhinology, Sinus and Skull Base Surgery, University Hospitals – Case Western Reserve University, 11000 Euclid Avenue, Cleveland, OH 44106, USA; [c] Section of Rhinology, Sinus and Skull Base Surgery, Head and Neck Institute, Cleveland Clinic, 9500 Euclid Avenue, A71, Cleveland, OH 44195, USA; [d] Minimally Invasive Cranial Base and Pituitary Surgery Program, Section of Rhinology, Sinus and Skull Base Surgery, Head and Neck Institute, Rosa Ella Burkhardt Brain Tumor Center, Cleveland Clinic, 9500 Euclid Avenue, A71, Cleveland, OH 44195, USA; [e] Minimally Invasive Cranial Base and Pituitary Surgery Program, Section of Rhinology, Sinus and Skull Base Surgery, Head and Neck Institute, Rosa Ella Burkhardt Brain Tumor Center, Cleveland Clinic, 9500 Euclid Avenue, S73, Cleveland, OH 44195, USA
* Corresponding author.
E-mail address: sindwar@ccf.org

Otolaryngol Clin N Am 50 (2017) 643–653
http://dx.doi.org/10.1016/j.otc.2017.01.015
0030-6665/17/© 2017 Elsevier Inc. All rights reserved.
oto.theclinics.com

INTRODUCTION

Endoscopic skull base techniques have advanced greatly over the years owing to various technological advances, including angled endoscopes, high-definition monitors, frameless navigation systems, high-resolution imaging, and improved anatomic knowledge. Perhaps the greatest innovations in endoscopic skull base surgery have come in the treatment of complex skull base defects and cerebrospinal fluid (CSF) leaks. Effective watertight repair of complex defects after skull base tumor resection emerged as the primary limitation to the endoscopic resection of advanced disorders. Thus, the ability to effectively reconstruct defects in this area represents a pivotal step in the ability to pursue endonasal endoscopic approaches. Over the past decade there have been considerable advances in the ability to reconstitute the separation between the intracranial and sinonasal compartments after endonasal skull base surgery. This article explores the methods and the materials used to accomplish skull base repair, discusses the indications for their use, and reviews the outcomes as reflected in the current literature.

ENDOSCOPIC SKULL BASE RECONSTRUCTION

Surgical treatment of skull base lesions of all types can be thought of as comprising 3 parts: approach, resection, and reconstruction. Endoscopy has provided an innovative, minimally invasive approach to various disease processes, but adoption was hampered by higher rates of CSF leaks. However, for endoscopic skull base surgeons, multiple methods developed over the last decade have assisted in providing the ability to improve outcomes and decrease leak rates. Modern repair processes include synthetic absorbable sealants and glues, synthetic dural replacement grafts, free autografts, vascularized flaps (both intranasal and extranasal), and free tissue transfer (**Table 1**). Although dependent on the type of CSF leak and type of defect, repair is typically accomplished using a multilayered closure using an underlay (subdural or epidural), an overlay graft or flap, and various types of intervening absorbable hemostatic agents (eg, cellulose, gelatin foam) alone or in combination with an absorbable glue or sealant.[1,2] The available options for repair are described here.

Free Autografts

Autografts, including free mucosa, fat, and fascia lata,[2] provided the first options for skull base reconstruction, and are still excellent options (**Table 2**). Fascia lata grafts are harvested from an incision (or 2 incisions with the less invasive technique) on the lateral thigh and offer a durable onlay material. The major drawbacks to the use of fascia lata are possible wound-related issues, especially in young physically active patients. The fat graft, typically involving abdominal adipose tissue, provides a suitable subdural inlay substance that is best used to fill large cavities left behind by resection

Table 1 Free autografts	
Local Grafts	**Remote Grafts**
Inferior turbinate mucosa	Fat (adipose)
Middle turbinate mucosa	Fascia lata
Septal mucosa	Bone (split calvarial)
Bone (vomer)	

or removal of tumor.[2] The two can be used in concert with a fat graft applied to the resection cavity and fascia lata placed over this secured with a packing and sealant.[2]

Alternatively, overlay materials can be harvested locally from the nasal cavity. Free mucosal grafts are obtained from the septum, inferior, or middle turbinates. The turbinate grafts are prepared by removing the turbinate and carefully stripping the mucosal tissue, and applied as an onlay repair (**Fig. 1**). Care is taken to ensure that the graft is then applied with the mucosal side out to prevent development of a mucocele.

Free bone grafts can be used when there is need for rigid repair. This need may occur in morbidly obese patients in whom there is potential for further brain or meningeal herniation over time.[1,3] These grafts can be harvested as split calvarial grafts or from the vomer and perpendicular plate of the ethmoid during septectomy.[1,4] The use of bone grafts is controversial because patients requiring postoperative radiation therapy may develop osteoradionecrosis and breakdown of the graft.[1,4]

Synthetic Dural Replacement Grafts

Inherent to the endoscopic approach to intracranial lesions is the need to open a layer of dura. This layer may be limited to the sella for trans-sellar approaches or involve more extensive opening of the dura (eg, diaphragma sellae, cribriform/planum dura, clival dura). The selection of the type or particular brand is left up to the surgeon; however, the grafts that can be sutured offer a sturdier repair substrate and are more pliant, making them easier to place and secure. Key to the use of these materials is the lack of additional donor site morbidity.

Intranasal Vascularized Flaps

The principal workhorse of contemporary endoscopic skull base repair techniques is the Hadad-Bassagasteguy flap, or the pedicled nasoseptal flap (NSF). First described in 2006,[5] it has proved to be a revolutionary development that vastly improved postoperative CSF leak rates.[2] As a result, there have been expansions in the types of lesions and locations accessible to endoscopic intervention. Some of the many properties that give the NSF its utility include consistent vascularity (superior septal artery terminal branch of internal maxillary artery), long and robust pedicle, ease of harvest, and customizability/adaptability.[4]

Typically, the inferior and middle turbinates are outfractured and a middle turbinectomy can be completed to facilitate harvesting the flap. As Hadad and colleagues[5]

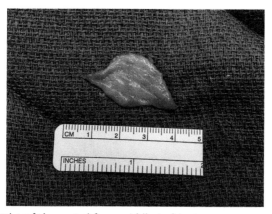

Fig. 1. Free mucosal graft harvested from middle turbinate.

Table 2 Vascularized flaps	
Intranasal Flaps	**Extranasal Flaps**
Posterior septal artery nasoseptal	Pericranial
Posterior pedicled inferior turbinate	Temporoparietal fascia
Posterior pedicled middle turbinate	Palatal
Bipedicled anterior septal	Occipital galeopericranial
Anterior inferior turbinate	Split calvarial osteopericranial
	Buccal fat pad
	Rotational temporal bone flap

described in their original article, the flap is made by making 3 cuts in the nasal septal mucosa using needle-tip monopolar cautery or cold techniques. The first superior cut starts along the sphenoid os and extends along the septum anteriorly, keeping 1 to 2 cm below the cribriform plate to preserve olfaction.[4,5] The second inferior cut starts from the superior margin of the choana, then extends across to the posterior margin of the vomer, then proceeds along the junction of the septum and the nasal floor over the maxillary crest. This inferior incision can be extended laterally to include the nasal floor and even the lateral nasal wall for coverage of wider defects, but care should be taken to avoid incising over the soft palate. The incision can be extended anteriorly as far as the junction between the septal mucosa and the vestibular skin. The two incisions are joined anteriorly by a vertical incision (**Fig. 2**). It is then carefully freed from the underlying bone/cartilage with care to preserve the posterior vascular pedicle. The flap is then tucked into the nasopharynx or maxillary sinus (**Fig. 3**) to avoid damage during the remainder of the operation (eg, tumor removal). The flap can be identified on

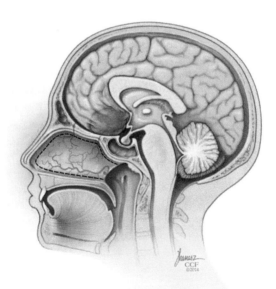

Fig. 2. Example of incisions made for a nasoseptal flap for repair following resection of the planum sphenoidale meningioma. (*Courtesy of* Cleveland Clinic Foundation, Cleveland, Ohio; with permission.)

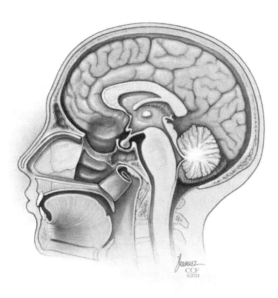

Fig. 3. Harvested nasoseptal flap tucked in the nasopharynx in anticipation of a planum sphenoidale defect following meningioma removal. (*Courtesy of* Cleveland Clinic Foundation, Cleveland, Ohio; with permission.)

postoperative MRI and should enhance with administration of contrast if the pedicle blood supply is intact (**Fig. 4**). At times, the NSF is not an option (eg, pedicle or blood supply interrupted from prior septoplasty, sinus surgery, or skull base surgery) and other local pedicled flaps must be considered.

The posterior pedicled inferior turbinate flap is one such option. It is best suited to sellar, suprasellar, and midclival defects considering the arc of rotation of the pedicle.[2,4] The blood supply originates from the inferior turbinate artery (a terminal branch of the posterior lateral nasal artery arising from the sphenopalatine artery).[2,4] The inferior turbinate can be medialized to facilitate harvesting the flap. The blood supply must be carefully delineated by first identifying the sphenopalatine artery as it leaves the sphenopalatine foramen. This blood supply is then followed to identify the posterior lateral nasal artery. Once this is done, 2 parallel incisions are made, superiorly as far rostral as the middle meatus and inferiorly along the medial margin of the inferior turbinate (and can be as far as the nasal floor to expand the flap's potential coverage), and a third vertical incision connecting the two. The flap is again carefully

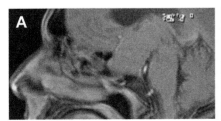
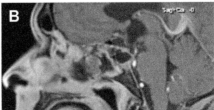

Fig. 4. Preoperative (*A*) and postoperative (*B*) MRI showing nasoseptal flap in place following resection of pituitary adenoma and repair of skull base defect.

freed, starting from the anterior tip and proceeding posteriorly with care to preserve the vascular pedicle. Because the blood supply can also invest the bone, some may need to be harvested with the flap. Bilateral flaps can be harvested, which is reported to provide coverage for approximately 60% of the anterior skull base.[1]

The posterior pedicled middle turbinate flap is another option that is best suited for limited defects of the planum sphenoidale, cribriform plate, sella, or some small clival defects.[2,4] This flap is limited by its small surface area, arc of coverage, and the technical difficulty in harvesting the flap. Anatomic variations including concha bullosa, paradoxic turbinate, and turbinate hypoplasia can serve to make flap harvest more challenging. However, it can be used as an alternative for the defects discussed earlier when the NSF is unavailable. The flap is supplied by a branch of the sphenopalatine artery at the posterior attachment of the turbinate. It is harvested using 2 incisions, with the first vertically along the anterior face of the middle turbinate head and the other horizontally along the attachment of the turbinate. It is then carefully freed in a superior to inferior direction with care to remove all bone from the undersurface. The flap is completed by sharp release of the inferior border, creating a posterior pedicle.

The posteriorly based NSF has been well described thus far; however, for very anterior defects of the cribriform or frontal sinus, other options often must be sought. The bipedicled anterior septal flap is based on the superior labial and nasopalatine arteries and is best suited for coverage of the frontal beak, posterior frontal table, and the anterior cribriform plate. It can also be used in the setting of revision surgeries in which NSF integrity is questionable.[4,6] The anterior inferior turbinate flap is based on a lateral nasal blood supply and is best suited to cribriform plate, frontal sinus posterior table (partial), and ethmoid roof reconstruction.[4,6] Both options can also be used in conjunction with the more traditional NSF for large or extensive skull base defects.

Although not common, these pedicled flaps can often be moved and reused, allowing a patient who has previously had an endonasal approach to a surgical site and now has a recurrence not to require another pedicled flap or morbid form of reconstruction.[7] It is essential to know the anatomy of the previous flap, and an endoscopic Doppler ultrasonography probe can be useful in this situation.

Extranasal Vascularized Flaps

Before the popularity of endoscopic techniques, open skull base techniques used multiple methods to repair skull base, dural defects, and CSF leaks. Many of these techniques have been adapted for usage in endoscopic surgeries. The endoscopic-assisted pericranial flap is one of these methods.[1–3,8,9] The pericranial flap blood supply is from the supraorbital and supratrochlear arteries. The flap is harvested by first making a 2-cm midline incision and a 1-cm lateral port incision along the coronal plane of the scalp. This step is followed by identification of the supraorbital and supratrochlear arteries using a Doppler, permitting demarcation of a 3-cm pedicle flap along the superior orbital rim. A subgaleal dissection is carefully performed from the posterior incisions to the level of the anterior pedicle. The flap is fashioned using monopolar cautery followed by elevation from the underlying calvarium. A transverse glabellar incision is then made of about 1 cm in length, followed by dissection off the underlying nasion. A subperiosteal plane is developed and extended superiorly to the pedicle of the flap. The flap is rotated into the nasal cavity using a bony conduit drilled through the nasion. Care should be exercised not to twist the flap as it enters intranasally and the dorsal aspect of the flap should be applied to the dural defect directly (as would occur in an open repair). Alternatively, a more traditional bicoronal incision can be made to facilitate harvest of the flap and avoid the potentially less cosmetic glabellar incision. The pericranial flap is best suited to defects anterior to the sella turcica.

The temporoparietal fascia flap has been used extensively in head and neck reconstructions and has also been adapted for endoscopic skull base repair.[2,4,8] It provides excellent tissue coverage and is a good option when there are limited intranasal options available. The flap is supplied by the superficial temporal artery (STA), which is a terminal branch of the external carotid artery. It can be harvested from either side of the scalp, but it is recommended to use the side ipsilateral to the skull base defect. The harvest begins with an anterior and posterior ethmoidectomy and a large maxillary antrostomy followed by clipping of the sphenopalatine artery and the posterior nasal artery at the level of the sphenopalatine foramen. The sphenopalatine artery is then dissected and followed, permitting exposure of the pterygopalatine fossa by removal of the posterior wall of the maxillary sinus. A portion of the lateral wall of the maxillary sinus is then removed, opening the infratemporal fossa and identifying the descending palatine artery. The contents of the pterygopalatine fossa are displaced inferiorly and laterally to expose the pterygoid plates. The pterygopalatine ganglion can be preserved by dividing the vidian nerve to permit displacement of the ganglion. The anterior pterygoid plates are reduced via high-speed drill, permitting a space large enough for tunneling the flap. A hemicoronal scalp incision can be made with care to preserve the STA within the subcutaneous tissue. The flap can be fashioned by incising the fascia laterally (the flap width can be determined based on the size or extent of the defect) followed by separation from the underlying muscle and deep fascia. The deep fascia is then incised and removed from the calvarial surface, permitting a passage for tunneling the flap. A lateral canthotomy incision is made to expose and separate the temporalis muscle from the lateral orbital wall and pterygomaxillary fissure, creating a tunnel that communicates the temporal fossa, infratemporal fossa, and the previously created transpterygoid approach.

The soft tissue tunnel is sequentially dilated by passage of a guidewire into the nose under endonasal endoscopic guidance and then advancement of percutaneous tracheotomy dilators over the wire. After an adequate tunnel is created, the dilators are removed, the flap is tied to the external end of the guidewire, and the nasal end of the guidewire is pulled out through the nostril, with the flap proceeding through the tunnel intranasally. The flap is assisted through the tunnel with external manipulation carefully to avoid rotation of the flap and to maintain its blood supply. The drawbacks of this method are that it necessitates a superficial incision, it places the frontotemporal branches of the facial nerve at increased risk, and it has a limited axis of rotation, limiting its application to clival and parasellar regions.[4]

There are several reconstructive options that have been well described in cadaveric models but are challenging in the clinical setting. The palatal flap has been described as an option of last resort.[1,4] It is supplied by the greater palatine artery and is elevated from the palate then passed through the greater palatine foramen. This option carries significant donor site morbidity and is currently not widely used. The pedicled facial buccinator flap has been suggested and studied in cadavers.[4] It is based on the facial artery, includes adjacent buccal soft tissue with or without muscle and mucosa, is passed through a maxillary window, and carries the risk of facial nerve and lacrimal damage. Likewise, the occipital galeopericranial flap is clinically challenging.[1,4] It is based on the occipital artery, necessitates release of neck muscles, and requires transposition through the pterygomaxillary space, maxillary antrostomy, posterior maxillectomy, and takedown of the inferior portion of the pterygoid plates. An adaptation of split calvarial osteopericranial flap was recently described in cadaveric studies and involves the endoscopic placement of the graft via a nasion-frontal osteotomy.[10] The use of the buccal fat pad was recently described as well and involves the endoscopic placement of a rotational flap, which is ideally suited for repair of large defects involving the greater sphenoid wing, inferior and superior clivus, sella, planum, and bilateral ethmoids.[8,11]

A vascularized rotational temporal bone flap was used for the repair of a large neuroendocrine carcinoma recurrence, as described by Zeiler and Kaufman.[12] These options are currently not favorable clinical tools and should be avoided in favor of more conventional and widespread options.

Free Tissue Transfer

Critical to the success of head and neck surgery has been the adoption of free tissue transfer by otolaryngologists. These same techniques can be used for significant defects of the skull base and tend to be used in the final rung of the reconstructive ladder. It is rare that any of these flaps are deployed in a purely endoscopic fashion, because insertion of this bulk of tissue generally demands larger exposures involving some type of open approach; moreover, flap anastomosis is performed microscopically through incisions over the typical recipient vessels (often the superior temporal or facial artery). The fine manipulation of the flaps may still be performed endoscopically, and, as can be imagined, it is far easier to move around tissue that is pliable, such as that seen with a radial forearm free flap or an anterolateral thigh flap, rather than the bone seen in a fibula free flap or a thick scapula free flap. Endoscopic access to the inferior aspect of these leaks is crucial to mitigate the depths of the defects created. This rung of the ladder is also extremely useful in patients who have sustained significant radiation to the midline skull base or those who have had multiple reconstructive efforts using lower rungs of the ladder.

Absorbable Sealants and Glues

Regardless of what repair options are selected, absorbable glues and sealants provide a critical adjunct to hold the multilayer repair sandwich together. A variety of options and methods exist but most frequently this is accomplished using dissolvable hemostatic agents or packing, coupled with an absorbable sealant.[2] Several commercially available options exist and most work well with the addition of an extended applicator to reach the repair site. The general approach to the application of glues and sealants, synthetic or otherwise, is to ensure that none of this resorbable material is placed underneath the graft that it is used to secure into place.

FRAMEWORK FOR SELECTION OF RECONSTRUCTION OPTIONS: A GRADUATED APPROACH

With the multitude of options available for reconstruction an effort has been made to define the indications and utility for each type of repair. A few essential factors help to dictate which types are suitable in a given situation. Probably the most important factor guiding the selection of a repair method is to classify the volume and flow of CSF leak (if any).[2] Visual inspection coupled with noting whether a ventricle or cistern was opened (ie, entrance into the intracranial space and arachnoidal dissection) help to define the flow type. The 3 basic CSF leak types can be classified as no leak (no intracranial opening, or visible leak), low flow (intracranial opening but minimal flow observed or no involvement of a cistern or ventricle), and high flow (intracranial opening, entrance into ventricle or cistern). When there is no CSF leak, the repair is at the surgeon's discretion and can range from simple epidural or subdural placement of a synthetic graft with packing and sealant, which can be augmented with the addition of a free mucosal graft or a similar autograft. Literature results show that nonvascularized grafts and vascular grafts are equally well suited for low-flow CSF leaks.[2] High-flow CSF leaks are best repaired using vascularized flaps and multilayer repair[2] (**Table 3**).

There are multiple independent factors that help to guide the decision-making process and that should also be considered. The extent of the skull base defect should be assessed because any surgery involving an extended approach (sella plus tuberculum sellae and planum sphenoidale) or the clivus should be repaired using a vascularized flap.[2,4] Specific disorders also carry an increased potential for postoperative leak and the use of a vascularized flap should be strongly considered. Among these disorders are meningiomas (extensive bony and dural resection with intracranial disruption of the arachnoid plane), craniopharyngiomas (often requiring expanded approaches and involving arachnoid dissection), Cushing disease (reduced healing from hypercortisolemia), and morbid obesity (possible increased intracranial pressure, also potentially present with Cushing disease).[2,4] Another factor that has been posited is the history of or need for future radiation therapy for the patient's disorder, because vascularized flaps are more likely to withstand the long-term effects of radiation therapy.[2] Likewise, patients who are undergoing revision surgery may also require vascularized flaps.[2,4]

Perioperative lumbar drain placement has not been shown to positively affect the postoperative leak rates when vascularized flaps are used, although high-quality evidence is lacking. However, lumbar drains have been shown to be effective as first-line therapy in postoperative leaks.[13]

The authors advocate a laddered approach to reconstruction whereby simple overlay repair with a free mucosal graft is used for uncomplicated low-flow CSF leaks, and the pedicled NSF is used as a workhorse for high-flow leaks. Moving up the ladder, when the NSF is unavailable, regional pedicled flaps (endoscopically harvested pericranial flap being our preference) or fascia lata are considered with the use of free tissue transfer as a last resort in rare refractory situations. Some centers routinely use the fascia lata graft more commonly in place of the NSF with good results. High quality studies comparing outcomes stratified by complexity of defect, disorder involved, and efficacy of different repair technique are currently lacking.

Table 3
Reconstructive ladder by cerebrospinal fluid leak type

No Leak	Low-Flow Leak	High-Flow Leak
Single layer	Multilayer	Multilayer
No repair	Autograft (fascia lata or mucosa)	Autograft (fascia lata or fat)
Autograft (fat or mucosa)	Synthetic dural replacement grafts	Synthetic dural replacement grafts[a]
Synthetic dural replacement grafts		Intranasal vascularized flaps
		Extranasal vascularized flaps
		Free tissue transfer[b]

Modifying factors (ie, factors that indicate need for a vascularized flap regardless of leak type): Cushing disease, morbid obesity, craniopharyngioma, meningioma, extended skull base approach, large defect, revision surgery, history of or future need for radiation treatment.
[a] If included as a part of a multilayer repair.
[b] If no vascularized flap is available/possible.

OUTCOMES

CSF leak repair outcomes for endoscopic endonasal approaches have been shown to be comparable with those of open repair procedures.[2] Soudry and colleagues[13] showed in a review that encompassed a total of 673 patients from 22 case series that the postoperative CSF leak rate was 8.5%, with a more recent literature review confirming a rate of 8.9%.[14–18] Patients who did not have an intraoperative leak had no postoperative leaks, independent of what repair method was used. Vascularized flaps had a success rate of 94% regardless of the materials used in conjunction with the flap (eg, free autograft). Free grafts achieved successful closure 82% of the time and the least successful repair involved fat graft with synthetic grafting as a subdural/epidural inlay with a success rate of 55%. The study also assessed the operative site/extent of the skull base defect. The anterior skull base was successfully closed 92% of the time overall, 67% to 93% with nonvascularized grafts, and 96% to 100% with vascularized flaps (nasoseptal or pericranial flaps). The overall success rate for sellar closures was 93%, with vascularized flaps achieving 94% to 100% success (both high-flow and low-flow leaks) with free grafts being successful 87% to 100% of the time for low-flow leaks alone. By far the most difficult site to close proved to be clival defects, with an overall success rate of 80%, a success rate of 60% for the single nonvascularized repair, and 100% for vascularized flaps.

Soudry and colleagues[13] were unable to completely define the role of perioperative CSF diversion (via lumbar drains) with this review. They did note that 38% of postoperative leaks were managed primarily with lumbar drain placement, whereas the remaining 62% required surgical repair with or without lumbar drain placement.

SUMMARY

Endoscopic endonasal approaches have attained a more prominent place in skull base surgery because of the expanding materials and technologies available for repair of CSF leaks and skull base defects. Multilayer approaches tend to be the most popular and durable solutions for CSF leaks. These approaches typically comprise a free graft or dural substitute placement (eg, fat graft with subdural/epidural synthetic graft placement) coupled with a free graft or vascularized flap onlay depending on the type of CSF leak encountered. Selection of the best repair method should be based on a laddered approach factoring in the specific factors, including the degree of intraoperative CSF leak, extent of skull base defect, specific disorder involved, and comorbidities present in each case. Using modern reconstructive methods, studies have shown that the postoperative leak rates for endoscopic repairs are comparable with those of open repair procedures. These advances have helped to make endoscopic skull base surgery a viable alternative to open procedures.

REFERENCES

1. Kim GG, Hang AX, Mitchell C, et al. Pedicled extranasal flaps in skull base reconstruction. Adv Otorhinolaryngol 2013;74:71–80.
2. Zanation AM, Thorp BD, Parmar P, et al. Reconstructive options for endoscopic skull base surgery. Otolaryngol Clin North Am 2011;44(5):1201–22.
3. Zuniga MG, Turner JH, Chandra RK. Updates in anterior skull base reconstruction. Curr Opin Otolaryngol Head Neck Surg 2016;24:75–82.
4. Clavenna MJ, Turner JH, Chandra RK. Pedicled flaps in endoscopic skull base reconstruction: review of current techniques. Curr Opin Otolaryngol Head Neck Surg 2015;23:71–7.

5. Hadad G, Bassagasteguy L, Carrau RL, et al. A novel reconstructive technique after endoscopic expanded endonasal approaches: vascular pedicle nasoseptal flap. Laryngoscope 2006;116:1882–6.
6. Meier JC, Bleier BS. Anteriorly based pedicled flaps for skull base reconstruction. Adv Otorhinolaryngol 2013;74:64–70.
7. Zanation AM, Carrau RL, Snyderman CH, et al. Nasoseptal flap takedown and reuse in revision endoscopic skull base reconstruction. Laryngoscope 2011; 121(1):42–6.
8. Hachem RA, Elkhatib A, Beer-Furlan A, et al. Reconstructive techniques in skull base surgery after resection of malignant lesions: a wide array of choices. Curr Opin Otolaryngol Head Neck Surg 2016;24:91–7.
9. Lal D, Cain RB. Updates in reconstruction of skull base defects. Curr Opin Otolaryngol Head Neck Surg 2014;22:419–28.
10. Engle RD, Butrymowicz A, Peris-Celda M, et al. Split-calvarial osteopericranial flap for reconstruction following endoscopic anterior resection of cranial base. Laryngoscope 2015;125:826–30.
11. Markey J, Benet A, El-Sayed IH. The endonasal endoscopic harvest and anatomy of the buccal fat pad flap for closure of skull base defects. Laryngoscope 2015; 125:2247–52.
12. Zeiler FA, Kaufmann AM. Vascularized rotational temporal bone flap for repair of anterior skull base defects: a novel operative technique. J Neurosurg 2015;8:1–4.
13. Soudry E, Turner JH, Nayak JV, et al. Endoscopic reconstruction of surgically created skull base defects: a systematic review. Otolaryngol Head Neck Surg 2014;150:730–8.
14. Borg A, Kirkman M, Choi D. Endoscopic endonasal anterior skull base surgery: a systematic review of complications over the past 65 years. World Neurosurg 2016;95:383–91.
15. Dehdashti AR, Ganna A, Karabatsou K, et al. Pituitary adenomas: early surgical results in 200 patients and comparison with previous microsurgical series. Neurosurgery 2008;62:1006–17.
16. Zhang M, Singh H, Almodovar-Mercado GJ, et al. Required reading: the most impactful articles in endoscopic endonasal skull base surgery. World Neurosurg 2016;92:499–512.e2.
17. Choby GW, Mattos JL, Hughes MA, et al. Delayed nasoseptal flaps for endoscopic skull base reconstruction: proof of concept and evaluation of outcomes. Otolaryngol Head Neck Surg 2015;152:255–9.
18. Thorp BD, Sreenath SB, Ebert CS, et al. Endoscopic skull base reconstruction: a review and clinical case series of 152 vascularized flaps used for surgical skull base defects in the setting of intraoperative cerebrospinal fluid leak. Neurosurg Focus 2014;37(4):E4, 1–7.

The Operating Room of the Future Versus the Future of the Operating Room

Amin B. Kassam, MD*, Richard A. Rovin, MD, Sarika Walia, MD,
Srikant Chakravarthi, MD, Juanita Celix, MD,
Jonathan Jennings, MD, Sammy Khalili, MD, Lior Gonen, MD,
Alejandro Monroy-Sosa, MD, Melanie B. Fukui, MD

KEYWORDS

- Integrated system • Informatics • Neuronavigation • Tractography
- Corridor surgery • Cellular imaging • Robotics • Iterative learning

KEY POINTS

- The operating room of the future will be an informatics-driven platform.
- The information will be collected seamlessly in the background and provide for iterative learning.
- The information must be available in real time.
- Quality assessment and planning are integral features in informatics-based patient care.
- Advanced robotic optical imaging in synergy with real-time, integrated imaging can potentially reduce risk associated with surgery.
- Patient-centered cellular informatics in association with this operative paradigm will be the future of targeted therapy, which will occur *in situ* to restore the state of health.

 Video content accompanies this article at http://www.oto.theclinics.com.

INTRODUCTION

The art of surgery has evolved dramatically over centuries in hopes of progressively becoming a science. Its precision will continue to evolve and refine as critical knowledge is acquired, curated, and shared, to develop predictive and iterative patterns of learning, thereby delivering the fundamental requirements to minimize variance and enhance safety. By way of analogy, the aeronautic industry has been subject to the

Disclaimer: Please note that any opinions, findings, and/or conclusions expressed in this body of work are those of the author(s) and do not reflect the views of the above mentioned companies.
Disclosures: A.B. Kassam serves as a consultant for (1) Synaptive Medical Corporation, (2) KLS Martin Corporation, (3) Medical Advisory Board for Medtronic Corporation. J. Celix, S. Walia, S. Chakravarthi, J. Jennings, S. Khalili, M. Corsten, R.A. Rovin, and M.B. Fukui have nothing to disclose.
St. Luke's Medical Center, Aurora Neuroscience Innovation Institute, 2801 West Kinnickinnic River Parkway, Suite 630, Milwaukee, WI 53215, USA
* Corresponding author.
E-mail address: amin.kassam@aurora.org

Otolaryngol Clin N Am 50 (2017) 655–671
http://dx.doi.org/10.1016/j.otc.2017.01.016
0030-6665/17/© 2017 Elsevier Inc. All rights reserved.
oto.theclinics.com

Abbreviations	
CS-m	Conventional stereoscopic microscope
CT	Computed tomography
CTA	Computed tomography angiography
3D	Three dimensional
DoF	Depth of field
DTI	Diffusion tensor imaging
FoV	Field of view
HD	High-definition
NA	Numerical aperture
ROVOT-m	Robotically operated video telescopic microscope
VoV	Volume of view
VT-m	Video telescopic microscopy

same evolutionary process, and there is much to be learned from it. Much like in medicine, the individual patients' frustrations have remarkable similarities to passenger service frustrations, such as unanticipated events, delays, circumstances (eg, weather), escalating costs, and growing bureaucracy.

However, a key difference when comparing the patient-passenger paradigm is the overall safety profile. The incidence of airline crashes relative to the number people transported shows a remarkable safety record across multiple pilots, multiple airlines, and multiple countries, resulting in minimal variance and remarkable safety.[1,2] In comparison, the variance in surgery can be significant. However, unlike the airline industry, the mechanisms to quantitate and report such variances remains primitive. As the era of the risk-and-reward economy in medicine begins, this is bound to change. Rather than being financially rewarded for crashes (complications) that lead to more billable procedures, clinicians will now be economically penalized as they transition to a risk-shared economy. So what does this mean for the future of the operating room (OR)?

A period of transformative change is beginning, much like the airline industry experienced decades ago. The initial efforts to fly with minimal instruments and undertake uncoordinated exploratory routes without critical preflight and intraflight information were replaced when the high risk of catastrophic events was realized. The economic implications of a single crash and loss of lives became apparent and paramount in creating strategies that mitigated the exorbitant human and economic costs. To look past the human elements, how many seats would have to be filled and purchased to pay for the financial costs associated with a single crash? This provided key motivation to develop both technology and integrated processes to mitigate risk by creating a high-reliability system (**Fig. 1**). The art of flying evolved rapidly into a precise aeronautic science that has become inherently and inexorably dependent on the knowledge that is acquired, curated, and shared to develop predictive patterns to facilitate iterative learning. The very act of a crash is objectively captured and carefully scrutinized in the black box to provide for iterative learning.

As medicine enters an era in which risk is of paramount concern, the same evolution is anticipated to occur. As such, the OR of the future is rapidly transitioning from an exploratory, experiential learning environment (the art of surgery) to an information-driven, iterative learning environment with incremental precision and predictive learning. Explicitly, the authors believe the future OR to be a vital hub of real-time physiologic, anatomic, and pathologic tissue interrogation that is contemporaneously and seamlessly collected in the background, much like the manner in which the e-commerce collects our individual consumer habits to design precision marketing to acquire and curate critical information, then act on it without the consumers leaving their homes.

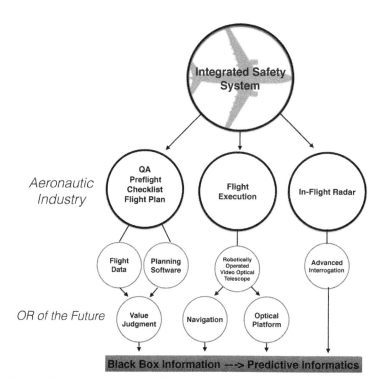

Fig. 1. The architecture of the OR of the future patterned after the aeronautic industry. Phase I for both industries requires sequential quality assessment, preflight checklist, and trajectory flight plan, and is then subject to value judgment. Phase II constitutes the flight plan and execution, with synthesizing navigation, robotics, and an advanced optical platform. Phase III comprises in-flight (*in situ*) radar accomplished with advanced imaging to interrogate at the cellular level. Ultimately, the background collection and analysis of data acquired during these 3 phases through intelligent informatics will provide the substrate for an augmented, predictive platform. QA, quality assurance.

The aeronautic industry has shown that, in order to transform this information into useful knowledge that can minimize variance and enhance safety, several key requirements must be met the key OR functions and the aeronautic correlations are provided below: (see **Fig. 1**):

1. The information must be quality assured:
   a. Information such as flight traffic patterns must *a priori* be subject to rigorous quality checks before any interpretation and before being used for decision making
   b. Flight traffic must be accurately collected to generate reliable flight plans
2. It must be acquired and delivered at the point of intervention in real time:
   a. Information from the tower must be provided in real time to the cockpit
3. It must be delivered in a user-friendly manner with as much automation balancing accuracy, eliminating human error, and data integrity as feasible:
   a. Flight plans are autopopulated
4. The systems must be fully integrated and nonsiloed:
   a. The navigation and autopilot systems are of the same platform
   b. Minimize the need for vendor interoperability

5. The system must have advanced, on-board interrogation platforms:
   a. Radar and other modalities to interrogate in real time potential variances that may affect the flight plan
6. Multimodality real-time data integration with the instruments or devices representing objective truth sources:
   a. The altitude is an objective measurement that is provided by the instrument rather than a subjective assessment by the pilot
7. A background informatics system that concurrently captures this information to create adaptive precision responses based on probabilistic predictive patterns and also curates the information to facilitate iterative learning, providing a substrate for intervention
   a. Autopilot function for adaptive responses subject to human governance
   b. Black box for curation
8. Rapid global information dissemination that links cause and effect, thereby facilitating iterative learning

PHASE I: QUALITY ASSESSMENT, PREFLIGHT CHECKLIST, AND FLIGHT PLAN

When applying these principles to define the skull base OR of the future, there are striking similarities that predict the evolution of what the future of the OR will look like (see **Fig. 1**; **Fig. 2**, Video 1). At present, there is little to no quality assessment of the imaging data that is acquired in radiology (representing the air traffic tower) and then provided to the OR; despite the significant variance in the images provided, they are often used for critical decision making. The air traffic controllers (ie, neuroradiologists) are located remotely, and nowhere near the runway. The authors believed that this needed fundamental restructuring and have already effected change in our practice, so that the future (our current) OR more closely mirrors the underlying architecture of the aeronautic

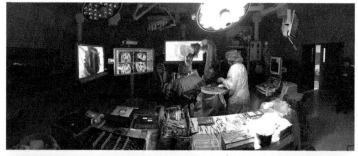

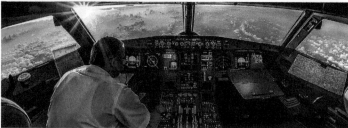

Fig. 2. The cockpit. The cockpit of an airplane is juxtaposed to the cockpit of our current OR, highlighting the vast amount of data that are provided in real time simultaneously to both operators and all personnel. This setup ensures that all operators receive the same information to support the critical decision-making process.

industry. Image variance, both in prescribing and execution, is an all-too-common phenomenon in surgery. We are convinced that automated software will be used to predict the correct imaging needed, based on specific anatomic requirements for the procedure and confirm, in an automated fashion, its quality-assured execution. Like the aeronautic industry, the multimodality imaging data, analogous to air traffic, will be thoroughly quality assured before being used in any capacity, and this will be a key risk mitigation strategy. In the aeronautic industry, detailed planning, with accurate target identification and trajectory planning, always precedes takeoff. This function is performed primarily by air traffic control and the navigators undertake the original planning, with validation and execution undertaken by the pilot. We have adopted this model by co-locating our neuroradiologist adjacent to the OR in a suite where similar flight plans by competency experts are created in mutual collaboration. This function is performed as a team with the radiologist providing details and imaging nuances in real time, at the point of care, adjacent to or in the OR, requiring that financial barriers to collaboration are eliminated in the interest of patient safety and risk mitigation. This system allows the neuroradiologist to function as a real-time clinician, providing competency expertise in image interpretation that is contextually relevant, and therefore valuable to the patient at the point of intervention; that is, on the runway and in flight.

We believe that skull base imaging constitutes 3 primary anatomic considerations:

1. Osseous framework:
   - Can usually be drilled and corridors created
2. Vascular:
   - Can usually be moved and, if needed, reconstructed or rerouted
3. Cranial nerves and white matter:
   - We consider the intrinsic white matter to be endophytic (as opposed to exophytic) nerves
   - Manipulation of both should be avoided

The layered consideration of imaging modalities (bone algorithm computed tomography [CT], CT angiography [CTA], three-dimensional [3D] structural MRI [**Fig. 3**], and 3D white matter tractography) mirrors the history of advances in skull base surgery. Just as instrumentation incrementally increased the safety profile of the aerospace industry, so did detailed imaging and optics herald the advances in skull base surgery. From our perspective, the first era of skull base surgery constituted exploratory flights. Initially, the main consideration was the technical ability to drill and disarticulate bone in order to gain access to disease, as shown on CT. This ability, coupled with the increasing familiarity with advances in optical instrumentation, allowed the emergence of the vascular era of skull base surgery. The operative microscope permitted the development of microvascular techniques that allowed vessels to be mobilized, rerouted, and reconstructed to further advance access to cranial base disorders.[3,4] With the advent of CT and CTA, vessels could be preoperatively assessed in relation to osseous landmarks, which allowed more detailed preoperative planning. At this point, the goal of complete resection admittedly outweighed that of preservation of cranial nerves and white matter function.[5,6]

With the development of effective radiosurgical and medical therapies, and the evolution of minimally invasive corridor-driven skull base surgery, the goals of resection changed to preserve neurologic function and quality of life, which are now well recognized to influence prognosis.[7] This mandate to preserve cranial nerve function ushered in a new era in skull base surgery that established a new paradigm in which the relationship of disease to cranial nerves essentially dictated the corridor, explicitly the evolution of 360° skull base surgery[8] (see **Fig. 3**). The directive to preserve neurologic function and, hence, quality of life resulted in a new edict: avoid crossing the plane of

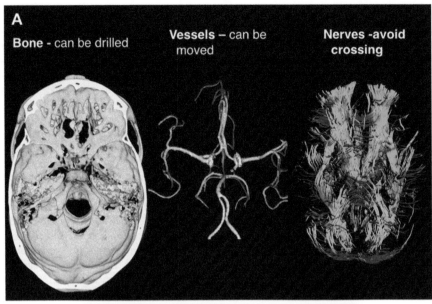

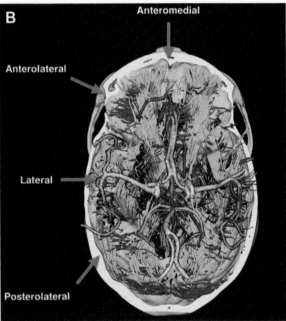

Fig. 3. Three-dimensional layering of osseous, vascular, and tractography data sets. (*A*) Three-dimensional reconstruction of (*left to right*) osseous CT layer, 3D vascular reconstruction of CTA layer, and 3D tractography layer. (*B*) All 3 layers have been combined in order to show the detailed anatomy to be considered and modeled in preflight planning in order to decide on the flight plan and create the safest operative trajectory.

cranial nerves. Loss of cranial nerve function has proved to be the most important and most common long-term morbidity that adversely affects quality of life.[8]

Preoperative imaging relied on MRI sequences that showed the cranial nerves as conspicuously as possible, and with as much contrast, including high resolution

T2-weighted sequences. However, the CT, CTA, and MRI had to be evaluated separately and essentially merged by the surgeon to create a map in order to determine the safest route to the target. This merger or fusion became semiautomated, but did so with minimal regard as to the quality of the initial data sets and image variance. The recent development of diffusion tensor imaging (DTI) has allowed access to an entire 3D map of the white matter of the brain (comparable with Google Street View), which, in the process, has created further challenges with this fusion of information. In addition to the sheer volume of white matter and cranial nerve data, the complex volumetric algorithms from which they are acquired result in profound barriers that have to be overcome to ensure accurate geometric fit and resolve warp correction. However, without postprocessing for 3D rendering, the tracts are simply displayed in two dimensions as colors indicating their primary orientation (red = transverse; blue = craniocaudal; green = anterior-posterior; **Fig. 4**). Using only that information to generate a safe corridor would be analogous to a pilot flying with no more route information than north-south, east-west, and altitude. The 3D rendering of the tracts is typically labor intensive and requires a neuroradiologist or surgeon to accomplish the hand-seeding of individual tracts. This method is analogous to mapping flight plans by hand, using the stars to navigate.

In the neurosurgical OR of the future, coregistration of high-quality, multimodality imaging incorporating CT and CTA (Video 2) with white matter tract mapping, and conspicuous cranial nerve dynamic 3D rendering, occur in real time using planning software (**Fig. 5**). This planning software integrated into a single platform can be used intraoperatively to create real-time simulation (**Fig. 6**). The software allows the team to develop and design a plan that can be fully processed and ready for

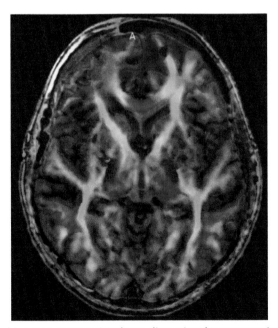

Fig. 4. Red-green-blue map. Conventional two-dimensional postprocessing of DTI data displays information regarding directionality of white matter tracts by encoding tracts in the transverse direction as red (commissural fibers), anterior-posterior direction as green (primarily association fibers), and craniocaudal direction as blue (primarily projection fibers).

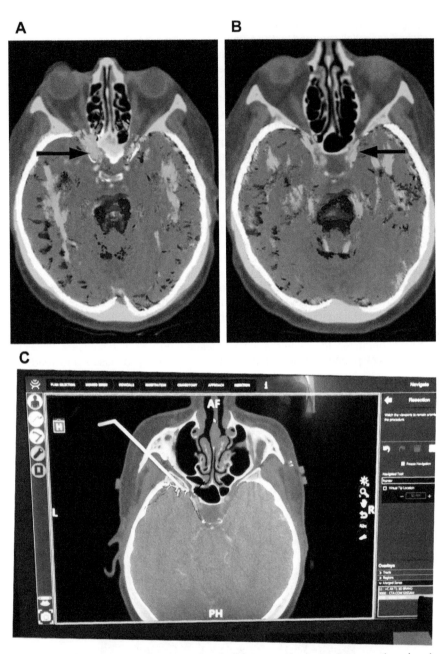

662 Kassam et al

Fig. 5. Anterolateral approach to anterior skull base meningioma. Preoperative planning and intraoperative execution during the orbitotomy show tractography coregistered with CTA with localization of the optic nerves (*A*) (*arrow*) and oculomotor nerves (*B*, green fibers) (*arrow*). The orbitotomy is cut to the level of the superior orbital fissure and respects the plane of the cranial nerves constrained within (*C*) (*arrow*).

A

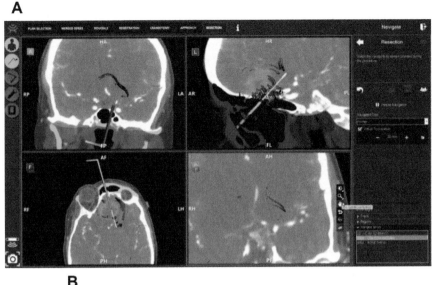

B

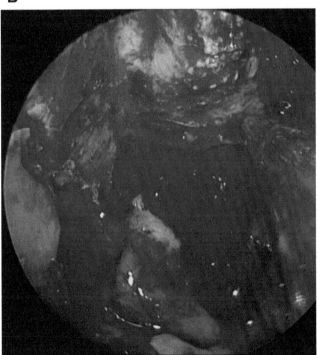

Fig. 6. Anteromedial, endoscopic approach to olfactory groove meningioma. (*A*) Real-time, intraoperative navigation during expanded endoscopic endonasal approach shows tractography in coronal, axial, sagittal, and endoscopic trajectory planes, coregistered to CTA (*A*; *top row*) and corresponding endoscopic view (*A*; *bottom row*). Intraoperative navigation display shows the tip of the navigation probe (*blue line*) inferior to the fovea ethmoidalis, pointing to left posterolateral tumor margin with the yellow line showing the depth from the probe tip to the fibers of the left IFOF. (*B*) Endoscopic view corresponding with the navigation images (*A*). IFOF, inferior fronto-occipital fasciculus.

execution in 15 minutes (Videos 3 and 4). The surgical planning system of the future provides automatically postprocessed 3D rendering of white matter tractography using substrate information that has undergone quality assurance, which is critical, given that planning is only as reliable as the imaging data from which it is derived (see Video 3). Just as the aerospace industry ensures safety through reliability, the planning software first subjects the imaging data to a rigorous quality review, ensuring that the imaging is of sufficient quality, and therefore reliable, before planning (see **Fig. 1**).

Next, quality-assured 3D tractography is coregistered to structural MRI sequences as well as with non-MRI data sets, including CT and CTA. The planning software allows sequential layering of bone algorithm CT, CTA, MRI, and 3D-rendered tractography data sets (see Video 2 and 4). The surgical team can analyze the detailed osseous, vascular, soft tissue, and neural anatomy serially and in layered fashion to study their interrelationships (Video 5). The synthesized data set permit evaluation of the relationship of exophytic cranial nerves and endophytic white matter tracts that primarily drive the surgical corridor choice to the targeted disorder along with vascular and osseous landmarks. The availability of quality-assured white matter tract and cranial nerve tractography, which can be reassessed in real time and intraoperatively in relation to unshifting osseous landmarks, increases their conspicuity to the surgeon, creating a new form of intraoperative instrument panel that should promote neural tissue preservation techniques (see **Figs. 5** and **6**; **Fig. 7**). With the surgeons now able to process the merged data, they are ready to "fly" through the surgical space with autopilot functionality and reliability, as well as to have the freedom to adjust the plan while in flight, if obstacles arise for which deviation is necessary.

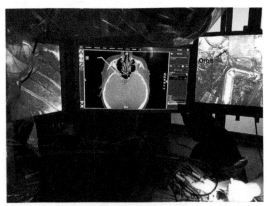

Fig. 7. The new operative instrument panel. Real-time panorama of instrument panel currently in our OR showing high-definition (HD) monitors that enhance magnification and resolution. The navigation panel (center) is simultaneously viewed along with the operative field (peripheral panels). The navigation probe placed on the sphenoid triangle at the margin of the superior orbital fissure during an orbitotomy shows the fibers of the third nerve as rendered with tractography, coregistered to CT, and allows the surgeon and cosurgeon to confirm or modify the flight plan during surgery. The coregistered CT/CTA/MRI/tractography can be reassessed in real time so that the surgeon can simultaneously cross-reference and recalibrate the surgical volume of view (VoV) with coregistered tractography and multimodality structural imaging. In addition, the HD display component of the optical chain offers a complete view of the surgery for all participants in the OR for a complete learning experience.

PHASE II: FLIGHT EXECUTION

The quest to enhance and optimize the ability to visualize surgical anatomy has seen tremendous evolution and advancement in the constituents of the optical system. The components of the optical system, referred to as the optical chain, comprise (1) the optical payload, (2) the light source, (3) the camera, (4) the holder, and (5) the display (**Fig. 8**). Following the inception of the original optical chain in 1876,[3] consisting of loupe magnification, an external light source, and the surgeon's head and neck as a holder and positional system, the next significant evolution did not occur for nearly another century. Over the ensuing 90 years, the system eventually evolved into the conventional stereoscopic microscope (CS-m) platform. When the CS-m was first introduced to neurosurgery in 1968,[4] it provided users with a far superior visual intraoperative experience. This improvement was especially important in the context of visualizing intrinsic, deep-seated neural and cerebrovascular structures, which enabled luminaries, such as Professor Rhoton, to eloquently unlock the mystery of the anatomy of the skull base.

Specifically, the large numerical aperture (NA) of the CS-m accepts light from a wide angle, converging and refracting it to a focal point, thereby providing high central resolution. However, the large NA, and associated significant bending of light, in turn creates spectral and optical distortions at the periphery, away from this central point of focus. This lateral distortion is directly proportional to the degree of magnification, resulting in a central focal point of a highly resolvable image with blurring and obscuration of the viewable, but unresolvable, peripheral field of view (FoV). The lateral distortion not only causes blurring but also may affect color, potentially creating chromatic aberration, which has the risk of changing the quality of the native image.

In summary, as the magnification is adjusted, it directly influences what can be seen centrally (useable/resolvable) and peripherally (just viewable and not resolvable). The FoV describes the area of the image that is viewable (x, y) and when the z-axis (ie, depth of field [DoF]) is added to this it converts the area to a volume of view (VoV). The same principles affecting FoV apply to the DoF, with a proportional reduction directly contingent on magnification. The greater the magnification the smaller the DoF requiring constant manual readjustments to compensate. The authors consider the useable and in-focus VoV as the most critical optical metric responsible for the overall appreciation of surgical anatomy and this has been shown to be restricted with the CS-m.[9,10]

The implementation of the endoscope in surgery was intended to correct and alleviate some of the deficits that resulted from the large NA of the CS-m, in particular with regard to the blurred, distorted, and therefore unusable FoV.[11,12] This work led to the development of video-based telescopic (video telescopic microscopy [VT-m]) optical chains. The initial efforts coupled high-definition (HD) cameras with endoscopic optical payloads and the video-based display. The VT-m systems not only untethered the surgeon from the delivery system, but, more importantly, the reduced NA created less peripheral distortion by capturing and refracting light with greater parallelity as opposed to convergence. Although beyond the scope of this article, practically, this creates a larger FoV, creating a focal plane rather than a focal point. Although this ushered in an era of minimally invasive surgery, it proved to have clear limitations.

The smaller NA improved the resolvable FoV but came at the expense of a significant reduction in the DoF, or the z axis of the image. The critical impact of this on 3D perception was easily overcome in endonasal surgery by recovering the loss of DoF with dynamic intraoperative manual movement. Leveraging a superior FoV and improved

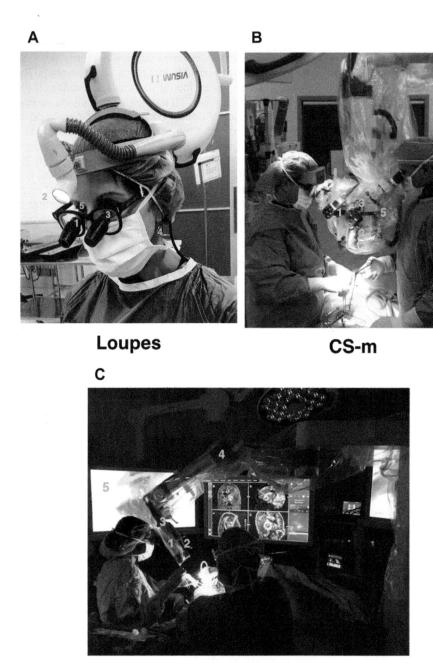

Fig. 8. Optical chain for each of the evolutionary surgical optical platforms. Loupes (*A*), conventional stereoscopic binocular microscopy (CS-m) (*B*), robotically operated video operative telescopic microscope (ROVOT-m) (*C*). The optical chain consists of 5 components: (1) optical payload; (2) light source; (3) camera; (4) holder; and (5) a display. (*Courtesy of* [*A*] Stryker, Kalamazoo, MI, with permission; and [*B*] Servo System, Synaptive Medical, Toronto, Canada, with permission.)

visualization with HD-coupled systems easily compensated for DoF, ushering in a new era of endonasal skull base surgery. However, the physics of endoscopic optics demanded dynamic movement, which is why the authors have been proponents of 2 surgeons working dynamically together, rather than relying on static holders.

This dynamic movement requires a cavity (air or fluid filled) that can afford unimpeded movement without risk of inadvertent injury to local structures, and therefore was seen as advantageous in the context of laparoscopy (ie, intracavitary thoracic or abdominal surgery) and endoscopic endonasal surgery.[11,13–16] However, this also explains why endoscopy has not penetrated intracranial surgery and has since been relegated to a secondary role. Explicitly, during intracranial surgery, movement within the parenchyma and anatomically rich cisterns can be hazardous. A case in point is posterior fossa surgery, in which surgeons are often reluctant to undertake dynamic movement in this anatomically dense and intricate region, particularly when there are blind areas with critical structures located proximal to the endoscope.

In order to combine the optical power and advantages of the CS-m and endoscope based VT-m systems, an optimized optical chain has recently been developed. This integrated optical chain takes each of the 5 components and leverages their individual attributes to create synergy in overall performance. This development has resulted in a novel and purpose-built exoscopic payload with an optimized NA and computer-machine interfaced robotic positioning system: the robotically operated video optical telescopic microscope (ROVOT-m) (Synaptive Medical Corporation, Toronto, Canada) (Videos 5–9).

Over the past year the authors have gained progressive experience with this optical chain and can report a substantial enhancement in the surgical environment visualized. We have recently undertaken a cadaveric and clinical study that will be the subject of a separate article, but we have been able to show both qualitative and quantitative differences in the visualization provided by the CS-m compared with the ROVOT-m. Specifically, by virtue of the optimized NA, any resulting degradation in resolution or light is easily recovered by enhancing other components of the optical chain (HD monitors, robotic optimal position, and enhanced camera). The synergy of these components yields an overall substantial improvement in the quality of the image with less peripheral distortion, less shadowing, and a truer native image in a larger and resolvable volume of view compared with the CS-m (**Figs. 9** and **10**).

The integration of this system's optical power, as well as the untethering of the operator, allows for 2 surgeons, a pilot and copilot, to work simultaneously and collaboratively with exactly the same view in focus for continuous decision-making support (see **Fig. 2**). This system also nets an immersive view for all participants in the cockpit of the OR, where the enriched view yields a full volume of view, facilitating greater engagement and knowledge sharing and thereby minimizing further risk. The preset, hands-free positioning capabilities track the surgeons' tools and thereby increase their surgical efficiency, allowing surgeons to focus on the surgery at hand rather than continuously adjusting the technology and, as a result, themselves. The improved ergonomics are likely to offer greater risk reduction by reducing surgeon fatigue.

PHASE III: THE FUTURE OF FLIGHT
Advanced Interrogation Systems

The next phase of the OR of the future is to focus at the cellular level through next-generation imaging that will allow advanced interrogation of normal and diseased neural tissue (degenerative and neoplastic), which will be systematically captured in the background, curated, and analyzed by the informatics system. As optical chains

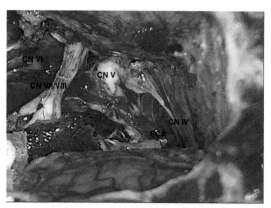

Fig. 9. The immersive surgical environment. Intraoperative view showing the cranial nerves (CNs) and arteries after resection of a glomus jugulare tumor along the skull base. Note that because of the increased immersive, useable and viewable VoV, CNs IV to VIII are simultaneously visualized in sharp focus and in full view exiting from the brainstem. The volume of view extends from the surface of the cerebellum to beyond the trigeminal nerve in depth and from the tentorium to the Dorello canal. SCA, superior cerebellar artery.

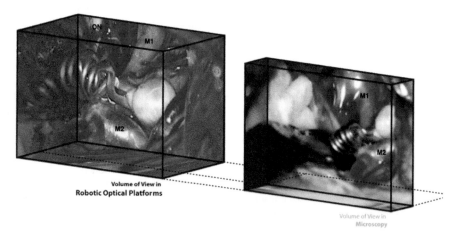

Fig. 10. Comparison of VoV between ROVOT-m and CS-m during clipping of a right middle cerebral artery aneurysm. The image on the right (CS-m) demonstrates, at high magnification, a good resolution of a relatively narrow focal point at the base of the aneurysm. While the remainder of the image is viewable, there still remains blurring and obscuration and a restricted depth of field. Note, in particular, the proximal M1. The image on the left (ROVOT-m) demonstrates a deeper field of view that is both viewable and useable. Again, note the resolution of the proximal M1 and distal M2 at the base of the aneurysm, all of which are resolvable. Every effort has been made to acquire both images at a similar magnification. In fact, the apparent magnification of the ROVOT-m is higher than CS-m. This is particularly important given that performance is better generally at a lower magnification for CS-m. (*From* Kassam AB, Corsten M, Curaudeau G, et al. First in Human Application of a Novel Integrated Image Guided Robotic Optical Telescopic Microscopy Positioning System: Cerebrovascular Surgical Applications. J Neurol Surg B 2016;77:A131; with permission.)

continue to evolve, the authors anticipate the ability to achieve real-time intracellular visualization with combined optical platforms providing *in vivo* chemical and structural contextual data. This information will be combined with *in situ* proton imaging, creating an entirely new paradigm for in vivo surgeons and pathologists. Surgeons will enter an era of true intracellular surgery in which detector robot systems will be the impetus behind a newly emerging generation of intracellular effector robotics, where increased levels of micro-visualization will allow for increased hand dexterity and micro-manipulation. As for neuropathologists, the authors anticipate the same evolution as occurred with neuroradiologists. Just as the function of neuroradiologists has been dramatically changed in this model to that of real-time clinicians, providing competency expertise in image interpretation that is contextually relevant and, therefore, valuable to patients at the point of intervention (ie, on the runway and in flight), pathologists will follow suit. These clinician-pathologists will use advanced interrogation tools to provide critical real-time information while the tissue is still in the patient to guide the surgical flight plan and execution.

For this to be realized there will be a need to continuously collect all data in the background to be integrated into a single system, again much like what has occurred in e-commerce industry. Initially, the story of a cell will follow it through the entire system from the OR to the bench and back, providing a continuous stream of data. The putative cell of origin will be targeted preoperatively, the specific flight plan to reach it with the least risk will be executed, the cell will be harvested and preserved as a living organ, and then the cell will be interrogated at a remote site in a recapitulated xenograft model. The data will then be extracted to benefit the donor organ.

A meningioma resected in the OR using this paradigm will have the progenitor cells targeted, captured, and remotely interrogated to provide a substrate for designing precision therapy (**Fig. 11**). At present, this requires remote interrogation and the creation of a xenograft animal model, with the human and mouse information fully integrated into one digital record. This record is projected and recorded in an overall sphere of informatics, and provides the ultimate patient-centric flight plan. This information, leveraged with technology and imaging, will create an interface that detects

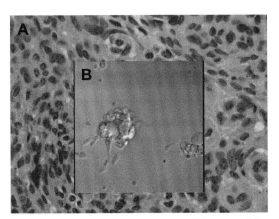

Fig. 11. Histopathology and cultured cells. Progenitor cell harvested from the right frontal meningioma resected in the OR. The larger background slide (*A*) shows the current state of histopathology, and the foreground (*B*) shows the cell culture. This cell culture is then interrogated with advanced imaging and the human-mouse complete data sets, including operative videos, harvest coordinates, and advanced interrogation linked into a single hierarchical data curation platform.

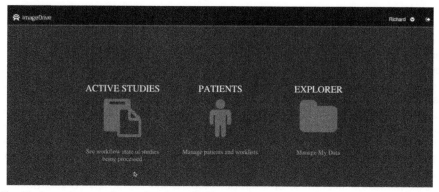

Fig. 12. ImageDrive. In future the OR, much like the aeronautic industry, will be a space where information is continuously and seamlessly gathered in an OR, allowing it to be beneficial on a global scale. In order for a black box (ImageDrive, Synaptive Medical, Toronto, Canada) of stored information to exist, quality assessment, planning, and quality control must be continuously enforced. Patient information will be captured and recorded with respect to definitive metrics. Development, acquisition, and storage of patient analytics will give rise to a future in which a patient's journey can be seen on a tangible interface for the further enhancement of the patient's care. (*Courtesy of* ImageDrive, Synaptive Medical, Toronto, Canada; with permission.)

and tracks individual patient patterns, spanning from preoperative imaging to the cellular level of the tumor. By automatically linking human-mouse information with same imaging interrogation platforms, quality-assured data are created that can be scaled at multiple levels. These data allow for scaled interrogation and intervention in multiple animals, and this in turn can be scaled to additional patients with similar conditions (similar flight plans and destinations). The safety and reliability of the predictive power will increase with increased flights and data captured from their black boxes (**Fig. 12**). This iterative learning will follow the same governing rules as the experience gained from the concept of 10,000 flight hours; that is, each transaction creates increased learning. The curation of the voluminous data aggregated and their input quality will be the primary determinant of the robustness of the predictive power generated by iterative analytics.

The next iteration of this paradigm will be to interrogate the cell without leaving the organ and based on informatics that affect real-time therapy. This *in situ* interrogation is analogous to using in-flight radar to course correct. The intermediate step of remote interrogation will be replaced with real-time *in situ* interrogation and intervention in the patient without the cell leaving the organ. This step will form the basis for the ultimate goal of precision-based cell therapy, including regenerative stem cell therapies, in which intracellular treatments for both pathologic and degenerative conditions will be the goal of surgery without leaving the organ in which they reside. In future the OR will be a venue that facilitates this real-time tissue interrogation, which, based on iterative learning and informatics, will then guide *in situ* therapeutics to restore the state of health.

ACKNOWLEDGMENTS

This article is based upon work that is supported by the following vendors:

1. Storz Corporation
2. Stryker Corporation
3. Synaptive Medical
4. Nico Corporation

Aurora Neuroscience Innovation Institute would like to acknowledge, and thank the above mentioned companies for their contributions in our Anatomic Laboratory.

SUPPLEMENTARY DATA

Supplementary video related to this article can be found at http://dx.doi.org/10.1016/j.otc.2017.01.016.

REFERENCES

1. Speers RD, McCulloch CA. Optimizing patient safety: can we learn from the airline industry? J Can Dent Assoc 2014;80:e37.
2. Rose NL. Fear of flying? Economic analysis of airline safety. J Econ Perspect 1992;6(2):75–94.
3. Kriss TC, Kriss VM. History of the operating microscope: from magnifying glass to microneurosurgery. Neurosurgery 1998;42(4):899–907 [discussion: 907–8].
4. Rand RW, Jannetta PJ. Micro-neurosurgery for aneurysms of the vertebral-basilar artery system. J Neurosurg 1967;27(4):330–5.
5. Berman JI, Berger MS, Chung S, et al. Accuracy of diffusion tensor magnetic resonance imaging tractography assessed using intraoperative subcortical stimulation mapping and magnetic source imaging. J Neurosurg 2007;107(3): 488–94. Available at: http://thejns.org/doi/full/10.3171/JNS-07/09/0488. Accessed December 10, 2015.
6. Abhinav K, Yeh F-C, Mansouri A, et al. High-definition fiber tractography for the evaluation of perilesional white matter tracts in high-grade glioma surgery. Neuro Oncol 2015;17(9):1199–209.
7. Pirris SM, Pollack IF, Snyderman CH, et al. Corridor surgery: the current paradigm for skull base surgery. Childs Nerv Syst 2007;23(4):377–84.
8. Kassam AB, Prevedello DM, Carrau RL, et al. Endoscopic endonasal skull base surgery: analysis of complications in the authors' initial 800 patients. J Neurosurg 2011;114(6):1544–68.
9. Botcherby EJ, Juskaitis R, Booth MJ, et al. Aberration-free optical refocusing in high numerical aperture microscopy. Opt Lett 2007;32(14):2007–9.
10. Watt SJ, Akeley K, Ernst MO, et al. Focus cues affect perceived depth. J Vis 2005;5(10):834–62.
11. Catapano D, Sloffer CA, Frank G, et al. Comparison between the microscope and endoscope in the direct endonasal extended transsphenoidal approach: anatomical study. J Neurosurg 2006;104(3):419–25.
12. Almeida JP, De Albuquerque LA, Dal Fabbro M, et al. Endoscopic skull base surgery: evaluation of current clinical outcomes. J Neurosurg Sci 2015. [Epub ahead of print].
13. de Lara D, Ditzel Filho LFS, Prevedello DM, et al. Endonasal endoscopic approaches to the paramedian skull base. World Neurosurg 2014;82(6 Suppl): S121–9.
14. Cuschieri A. Visual displays and visual perception in minimal access surgery. Semin Laparosc Surg 1995;2(3):209–14.
15. Jourdan IC, Dutson E, Garcia A, et al. Stereoscopic vision provides a significant advantage for precision robotic laparoscopy. Br J Surg 2004;91(7):879–85.
16. Vecchio R, MacFayden BV, Palazzo F. History of laparoscopic surgery. Panminerva Med 2000;42(1):87–90.

Index

Note: Page numbers of article titles are in **boldface** type.

Otolaryngol Clin N Am 50 (2017) 673–678
http://dx.doi.org/10.1016/S0030-6665(17)30076-2
0030-6665/17

oto.theclinics.com

Moving?

Make sure your subscription moves with you!

To notify us of your new address, find your **Clinics Account Number** (located on your mailing label above your name), and contact customer service at:

Email: journalscustomerservice-usa@elsevier.com

800-654-2452 (subscribers in the U.S. & Canada)
314-447-8871 (subscribers outside of the U.S. & Canada)

Fax number: 314-447-8029

Elsevier Health Sciences Division
Subscription Customer Service
3251 Riverport Lane
Maryland Heights, MO 63043

*To ensure uninterrupted delivery of your subscription, please notify us at least 4 weeks in advance of move.